RYAN A. MCPHERSON, D.O.

While You Were Asleep

*Behind the Scenes Stories from Residency at a Level 1
Trauma Center*

' "At a cardiac arrest, the first procedure is to take your own pulse."

—The House of God, 1978

Contents

Preface —The First Sunday of Spring

It was three-thirty in the afternoon on the first Sunday of spring. The weather was the nicest it had been in months. The sky was blue, the sun was shining, the air was crisp, flowers were blooming, and the birds were chirping gayly. It was a nice day. A perfect day.

I stepped through the doorway into the small consultation room that was tucked away in the emergency department. Behind me, crowding the doorway, was a young police officer and an even younger lady from the fire department crisis team wearing a green T-shirt and a look of concern on her face. At the far end of the small room, hunched over quietly on the couch with her dark hair covering her face, sat a distraught woman in her late fifties.

I edged closer and attempted to introduce myself, "I'm Dr.—" but before I could finish, the woman looked up and cut me off, "Is she dead?" She paused briefly, and before I could figure out what to say next, "Don't bullshit me," she said sternly, looking me straight in the eye.

The entire room was barely larger than a broom closet. There was a stiff, uncomfortable couch on which the woman sat, and next to it, two equally uncomfortable chairs with shiny wooden armrests. They were upholstered with an unrecognizable green vomit-colored pattern. Between them was a small table with a short lamp on it that contributed exactly none of the lighting to the room, all of which was provided by a blinding fluorescent fixture built into the ceiling. The walls were painted a sterile white, and one of them had a large, framed picture of an out-of-focus flower, a terrible stock

1

photo intended to induce calm and tranquility into those who looked at it. I gathered instantly that the woman didn't want to beat around the bush.

"Yes, she is dead," I said firmly and definitively, looking back at the woman, gauging her response.

"Who shot her?"

"I don't know."

Then, speaking quickly, the woman blurt out, "Did she have a gun with her? I know she did because she called me and told me she was going to buy a gun. Did the cops shoot her? Did they see her with the gun and shoot her? I bet the cops shot her."

"No, the police didn't shoot her," the young officer in the doorway cut in, uninvited.

No one else said anything.

Feeling like I had to say something, I reflexively used one of my standard lines, "I'm sorry to have to give you this news …" It worked, shattering the silence, but made nothing better.

She was hunched over again, her head in her hands, sobbing silently. I realized for the first time since entering the room that I was still standing, the conversation having started more abruptly than I had expected. They had warned us in medical school never to deliver important news while standing because it can be interpreted as condescending. Attempting to remedy my faux-pax I quickly sat down in one of the chairs near the woman and put my hand on her shoulder, trying to comfort her, but my hand on her shoulder wouldn't bring back her dead daughter. I knew it, and she knew it. My hand was only there to make me feel better. I felt the smallness of the room more than ever.

Suddenly, she looked up at me, a few strands of tear-soaked hair streaked across her face, "Can I see her?"

"Not yet," I said quietly, knowing this was not what she wanted to hear.

Raising her voice as she spoke, "I don't care what she looks like right now! Let me see her! She's my daughter!"

"The detectives need to do forensics first, then you can see her," the young officer cut in again.

"Why? Do you think someone else shot her? She shot herself, I know she did! She told me she was going to! Let me see her!" She was yelling now, desperate, her eyes darting between each of our faces, searching, hoping for one of us to relent and take her to her daughter.

"Let me introduce you to someone who can help. She's a grief counselor with the fire department," I said calmly, gesturing for the young lady in the green T-shirt to come in.

The young lady stepped through the doorway and into the room. I noticed for the first time that she was practically the same age as the woman's daughter. She moved carefully across the room and knelt down beside the woman, making herself eye level with her. She placed her hand on the woman's knee, and in a soothing voice, she said, "We are going to get through this."

The woman was hunched over again, crying quietly to herself. Silently, I got up and slipped out of the room unnoticed. My part was done. More of a formality than anything. The entire interaction had lasted less than a minute. There was no grace in telling a mother that her twenty-two-year-old daughter was dead. That less than thirty minutes ago she had been brought to the hospital with a hole in her head and her brain sliding down the front of her face. That she had driven to a gun store, bought a gun, bullets, and in broad daylight in the shopping center with everyone watching, pulled the trigger. No grace at all.

It was three-thirty-one in the afternoon on the first Sunday of spring. The weather was the nicest it had been in months. The sky was blue, the sun was shining, the air was crisp, flowers were blooming, and the birds were chirping gayly. It was a nice day. *Almost* a perfect day.

At first glance, it may seem like this book is not for everyone, but that assumption would be wrong. Although the stories are set against the backdrop of medicine, there is something in here for anyone who has ever felt like they didn't belong.

This is the story of my journey from a blood-phobic kid who couldn't focus on anything, to a trauma surgeon at a Level 1 trauma center. When you're in the hospital, you're having a horrible day. When I'm in the hospital, I'm at work. This book will take you behind the scenes to share the experiences of the people who take care of you, who make life or death decisions in the middle of the night for you, and who may one day have their hands inside of you.

The point of the stories in this book is not to shock or impress anyone, but simply to offer a look into the experience of medical and surgical trainees who spend every waking moment of their life dedicated to mastering the art of medicine and surgery.

Out of respect for people that were involved, and to protect the identity of patients, I have changed names and any details about them that may inadvertently reveal their identities.

Lastly, it should be noted that artificial intelligence (A.I.) such as ChatGPT, was not used to generate content, write, or edit this work.

CHAPTER 1—How It Started

It was a hot and dry autumn afternoon in Riverside, Southern California, and the sun was beating down on my head. I was in first grade, and my lips were chapped from the Santa Ana winds that had been blowing all week. With each gust of wind, dust lifted up off the playground, swirled around in the air, dancing, before finally falling back down onto the ground. I was on the far side of the playground with some friends playing on the monkey bars during afternoon recess when we heard a scream come from the direction of the school building. We stopped what we were doing and turned, shielding our eyes from the sun, and faced the school building. We saw teachers running toward the front, where the scream had come from. We couldn't tell what was going on from where we were, but we watched as kids and more teachers began to gather around something. Although I didn't know what had just happened, I could tell it was something bad. Despite the heat, hairs on my arms and back of my neck began to stand up.

After watching for several minutes, my friends began to grow frustrated that they couldn't tell what was going on. One of them, Joey, volunteered to walk over and see for himself. Not wanting to come off as wimps, the rest of us quickly said that we would go as well. We set off in the direction of the growing crowd of students, Joey eagerly in the front, and me, much less eagerly, in the back.

By the time we got to where the crowd had gathered, the teachers had been able to form a perimeter, holding back the students. We arrived at the back of the group, which was buzzing with chatter. Joey nudged one of the taller kids who was craning his neck over everyone else and asked him what had happened.

"One of the first graders fell off the bench and busted his head open!" he said excitedly, nearly shouting. "There's blood everywhere!"

A couple of the students around us who had overheard this all screamed "Eewww!" in unison and then giggled. It was the same type of immature "ew" as if they had witnessed a girl kiss a boy. They were unfazed. I was not. My stomach churned and my legs felt weak.

Despite this, I stayed. I didn't want my classmates to make fun of me later for running away. While my friends all stood on their tiptoes, trying to get a glimpse of the blood bath, I stared at the ground and pretended I was elsewhere. Still, I overheard updates as they were shouted through the crowd between the kids.

"I saw some of his brain come out!"

Eventually, the ambulance arrived, the first grader was taken away, and the crowd of students dispersed. My friends, all unfazed, had already moved on and were talking about the new *Jurassic Park* movie that was coming out. I, on the other hand, could not stop thinking about what had just happened. Not only was I disgusted and terrified, but I was also intensely curious. My mind was racing. I wondered what had happened to the kid. Did he die? Was it possible to survive cracking open your head and having some of your brain come out? If so, how did they fix it? What would the kid be like afterward, would he be different?

Despite my curiosity, terror won out. I was so terrified that for the rest of my time in elementary school, I would go out of my way to avoid that bench. From a distance, I even thought that I could see a stain on the ground from where his brain had spilled out.

I hoped that my discomfort with bodily functions would ago away as I got older. But still, whenever someone would vomit, other kids would laugh. They thought this was funny. Meanwhile, I would become extremely uncomfortable and would try not to vomit myself. In seventh grade, I narrowly avoided embarrassment and ridicule when this exact situation happened.

It was just after lunch, and I was sitting in history class trying to stay awake.

Next to me, I noticed that my friend Daniel had put his head down on his desk. I didn't think much of it, given the fact that it was a warm afternoon just after lunch, and at that time in my life, history was about as interesting as watching grass grow. I nudged him, trying to wake him up so that he wouldn't get in trouble, but he didn't move. I remember thinking to myself, jokingly, that he was probably in the middle of a really good dream.

Soon, the bell rang, indicating that class was over. There was a roar of noise as everyone stood up and immediately began talking, as we all prepared to move to our next class. Daniel, however, didn't move. Another classmate of mine, Aaron, saw him hunched over on his desk, and like me, thought he was still sleeping. We thought that this was pretty funny and began to laugh. Aaron started poking Daniel to try and rouse him, but nothing happened. Aaron and I joked that the history lecture had been so boring that it had put him into a deep sleep. We laughed even harder. Then, Aaron grabbed Daniel's shoulder and jerked his upper body upright. To our shock, Daniel's body was completely limp. His eyes were open but focused on nothing, and a thick stream of vomit ran from his mouth across the desk and onto the floor. Seeing this evoked sheer terror in me, and I ran.

I ran out of the room and down the hall. I had no idea where I was going. Out in the hallway, I paused for a moment to collect myself. I had no idea what I had just witnessed, or what was going on. I started running again until I burst into the school's front office, startling the secretary.

She looked up from her desk at me and lowered her glasses, "Can I help you?" she asked, with a hint of annoyance at being disturbed.

"Something is wrong with one of the kids in room 2A!" I shouted, breathlessly. "I think he's very sick!"

"And what is wrong with him?" she replied, impatiently.

"I don't know." I tried to explain what had just happened, but I couldn't think straight. "Asleep … not seeing … threw up." My fractured recollection of the events only confused and frustrated her further.

"Let's go look for ourselves then, shall we?" she said, as she stood up.

This did not sit well with me. The last place I wanted to go was back to the classroom. I was terrified of what I would see, but I trailed behind her—at least she would be a shield as we stepped through the doorway into room 2A.

Back in the classroom, Daniel had regained consciousness but was groggy. Our history teacher had cleaned up the vomit and was tending to him. I never once saw her hesitate. How could she be so fearless? The remainder of the class was still gathered around, whispering to each other.

Aaron noticed that I had returned to the classroom and asked me where I had gone. I just shrugged and told him it was none of his business. "Did you run away because you were scared?" he taunted.

How did he know!? I wondered, both shocked and embarrassed. I started to worry that other kids would overhear him and make fun of me also. I needed to make something up, and quickly. My mind raced, frantically searching for a plausible excuse for my sudden absence. Then I had the answer.

I informed him in a very matter of fact way, that while he had stood around ogling, I had gone in search of help, gesturing toward the secretary who was still standing nearby.

"Whew," I thought to myself, "months of ridicule and pranks averted."

Afterward, Daniel missed several days of school. There was a rumor going around that he'd had a seizure and needed surgery to remove a tumor in his brain. It wouldn't be until a decade later that I'd be able to put the pieces together and figure out that Daniel had had an uncommon pituitary tumor.

The first time I ever saw two people fight—I mean *really* fight—was when I was a freshman in high school. During lunch break, Eddy, one of the athletes, made fun of a necklace that another kid, Brian, was wearing. Instead of waiting for Eddy to get bored and move on, Brian shoved him in the chest. Eddy shoved back, so Brian shoved him again. Then their faces got really close to each other's, almost like they were about to kiss. Everyone immediately gathered around them, formed a circle, and began to chant, "Fight, fight, fight!"

Someone pointed out that the middle of the quad was not the ideal venue for a fist fight, so the whole crowd moved around to the less-visible back of the school. I have no idea why I went with them. Now, safely hidden behind the school, Eddy and Brian squared off. They both put their hands up in front of their faces and moved their feet like they were dancing. I was expecting some karate kicks like in the movies … but that was not what happened.

Almost immediately, Eddy quickly moved in and landed three huge blows across Brian's face. Blood shot out of Brian's face and splattered all over the wall of the school. Brian instantly fell to the ground, clutching his face. The crowd was screaming. Eddy raised his hand victoriously in the air, the one that he had struck Brian with, and then walked away into the crowd, leaving Brian behind on the ground, holding his head in his hands.

At that moment, I honestly believed Brian was going to die. I had never seen someone lose so much blood before in my life. It coated the side of the school like red paint. I looked down at Brian on the ground. I wanted to help him, but I didn't know how. I was too scared to even touch him. I felt helpless. Eventually the crowd dispersed, and to my utter disbelief, Brian was able to get up and walk away with them.

As I matured into high school, my main focus became skateboarding. It was all I cared about. My friends and I would spend every chance we had listening to punk rock and skateboarding at different locations around town, getting kicked out of them, and filming it all making *Jackass*-type skateboarding videos. Throughout this process, I got pretty beat up from falling down. I constantly had bruised shins and scraped elbows. But skateboarding did little to help with my discomfort around blood. Instead, my fear of blood became the foundation for a new anxiety, the feeling that I didn't belong amongst my peers, that I was an imposter.

When my friends and I weren't skateboarding, we were watching skateboarding videos. Every skateboarding video has a "spills" section where clips of the skateboarders falling down are shown. Sometimes they fall pretty hard. For a lot of my friends this was the best part of the video, and they would cheer, cringe, and make groaning noises with each fall. Meanwhile, I would quietly look away, considering the unimaginable pain and damage that each fall was causing the skater's body. At the time, there was a well-known skate video called "The Reason" which was rumored to have one of the gnarliest falls in it. Allegedly, one of the skaters fell grinding a handrail, splitting his head open, and bleeding everywhere. The camera man continued filming, even following him to the hospital. "Just like in elementary school," I thought to myself. I hadn't seen the video yet. I was too terrified. I had seen plenty of action movies with gore in them, but that was all fake, I told myself. This, on the other hand, was a documentary, it was real.

I avoided watching the video and asked my friends so many questions about that particular scene that they eventually grew suspicious. It didn't take long for them to figure out that I was afraid to watch it. From then on, every time we gathered to watch a skate video, they always joked that they were going to surprise me and put in that particular video and fast forward to that scene. This kept me on edge for a long time. (In the end, they never actually did it. Much later, when I was older, I finally did watch the video. The scene wasn't nearly as bad as I had anticipated after being built up in my mind for so long.)

As senior year of high school approached, it became clear that most of my friends were going to college. The main topic of conversation around the neighborhood became which big-name college or university my friends were going to attend. To put it mildly, I was not a great student. School had always just been something that you were supposed to do. While other students— through forceful encouragement from their helicopter parents—saw high school as a gateway to greater things, I had always treated it like something I didn't need to do well at—I just had to not fail. Despite being naturally athletic, I had avoided participating in team sports throughout high school. Most of them required staying after school for practice and showing up on weekends for games. That would have cut into my skateboarding and movie-making time, so I decided to pass. I had no extracurriculars to add to a college application.

My lack of ambition was obvious to my parents, who I'm sure had become very nervous around this time. Tony Hawk notwithstanding, they didn't see skateboarding as a viable career path. Because I spent more time watching skateboarding videos and listening to Blink-182 than I did taking AP classes, my friends' parents thought that I was a bad influence on their children. They made it clear they did not want their kids hanging out with me, for fear that I would derail their futures as well. Although it was never explicitly said, the message I received was: Success of any kind was not expected of me. Slowly, adults' lack of confidence in me began to erode my self-confidence, and I began to grow sort of comfortable with the idea that I might be a failure. By which, I mean as comfortable as someone wearing a rough wool sweater in July.

I suggested to my parents that maybe I shouldn't go to college, but this proposal was immediately shot down. Despite my disinterest in school, lack of AP classes, and dearth of extracurricular activities, I was never a *bad* student. Furthermore, much to everyone's surprise, I had done well on the SAT. I wound up with a modest scholarship to Whittier College, a small local liberal arts college in Southern California. The two most notable alumni are former president Richard Nixon, and Andrea Barber, the actress who played Kimmy Gibbler, the quirky next-door neighbor, on the '90s show *Full House*.

In order to help acclimate incoming freshman to living away from home for the first time, Whittier grouped new students together based on their declared majors. All of the art majors lived in one building, all of the science majors in another, and so on. Because housing was limited, incoming students were required to sign up as soon as possible in order to guarantee a spot living within the designated dorm for their declared major. In my truest fashion, I waited until the very last minute to do this.

I decided to declare myself a business major. By the time I signed up with the registrar, though, the dorms for business majors were, of course, already full. The only dorm available was Chemistry, so that's where I was placed. As a requirement for living in the chemistry dorm, I had to take science classes, including chemistry.

On my first day of college, after my parents had dropped me off, I set about the awkward task of making new friends. I started with the people in my immediate vicinity, the science majors. To my surprise, making friends wasn't so hard. I was the only non-science major among them. It became clear early on that most of them were studying science because they had their hearts set on medical school. Until six months prior, I had been seriously considering career paths that did not involve a formal education, so it was safe to say that I had never remotely considered med school. Besides, med school was only for the best and brightest, the cream of the crop, and all that bullshit. This was not how I thought of myself. The message everyone had worked so carefully to impress upon me—without ever having to say a word—remained carved into my brain and was now a part of my identity. I was not the best and the brightest, ergo med school was certainly not for me. That was fine with me, because I was queasy around blood … and nearly every other bodily function.

With each passing day, two things slowly began to shape the rest of my life: 1) I became bored with the required business classes for my major; I found my assigned science classes more engaging, especially biochemistry, and 2) All of my new friends that I was now living with, going to class with, studying with, eating with, and hanging out with, were dead set on going to med school. By the spring of freshman year, I was beginning to give med school a second thought—despite my nausea at the sight of bodily fluids.

My roommate, whose father was a physician, introduced me to the TV show *Scrubs*. Despite its popularity when it came out (2001-2010), I had never even heard of it. At that time, I had been busy watching *Rugrats* on Nickelodeon. I wasn't very interested in hearing him describe it to me, either. One day, he brought over a box set of DVDs and made me watch a marathon of episodes. I was quickly hooked. It never occurred to me that doctors could be *funny*. Or that a working in the hospital could be so interesting. I related to the show's main character J.D., who, in the pilot, was a first-year medical intern. He feared doing procedures on patients because, just like me, blood made him uncomfortable. Sure, it was just a TV show, but I began to feel that if J.D. could become a doctor, then so could I! I caved to peer pressure, dropped the business classes, and changed my major to biochemistry. Whoever said all peer pressure is bad?

People ask me all the time if I have ever seen *"insert name of popular medical TV show here."* Some I have seen and others I haven't. Most are extremely overdramatized and give an unrealistic impression of what practicing medicine is actually like. After finishing med school and residency, I rewatched *Scrubs*, and I must admit that *Scrubs* is by far the most accurate medical TV show I've seen. Not *ER*. Not *Grey's Anatomy*. Not even *House*. *Scrubs* does a great job of accurately capturing life as a resident, including the hospital hierarchy, what it's like to experience the loss of a patient, right down to the minutiae of day-to-day interactions. (Yes, including with the janitor.)

In the spring of my freshman year at Whittier, I decided to unveil my big change to my parents. I was in the car with my mom tagging along while she ran errands.

"I'm changing my major."

"Ok, to what?" she replied, without taking her eyes off the road.

"Biochemistry."

"Oh, that's fantastic! How come?"

"So I can get into medical school."

After a short pause, "You want to become a doctor?" She seemed puzzled, understandably.

"Well, uh, yeah, that's normally what people do when they go to med school," I stammered.

"But you've never wanted to become a doctor before."

"Now I do."

Cautiously, she proceeded. "Getting into med school is very difficult ..." she said, trailing off.

"I know," I replied, as I glanced out the window. I was growing irritated at her lack of confidence in me.

"Most people who become doctors start working toward going to medical school very early on, like in high school."

"I know," I replied tersely. Then I added, "I've been looking into it. I haven't closed any doors. If I change majors now, I can still meet the requirements to apply."

"Ok, but isn't there also a test you have to take as well to be admitted? The M- something?"

"Yes. The MCAT. Obviously, I'll have to study for it. I did OK on the SAT, I'm sure I can do well on this one too."

"Most people applying to medical school also do extracurricular activities."

My annoyance increased and my voice came out higher, tighter. "I *know*, and that's why I'm going to do community service and some other stuff too!"

Was she seriously trying to talk me *out* of trying to go to medical school? She was the one who wanted me to go to college in the first place. Most parents would kill for their kid to become a doctor. What was wrong with her? What was wrong with *me*?

We finished the drive home in silence. In retrospect, I shouldn't have been so surprised at her skepticism. Less than a year ago, the only anatomy I'd cared about was the parts of a skateboard. But I was determined to prove the doubters wrong. After years of rebellion via skateboarding, flaunting authority, and doing the opposite of what I was told, I was going to become a new kind of rebel. One who proved everyone else wrong by going to med school.

CHAPTER 2—The Interview

Despite my high score on the SAT, I didn't do well the first time I took the MCAT. This was a shock, because I believed I had a good understanding of the material. It was the summer between my junior and senior year of college, and I had chosen to spend my free time outdoors—going to the beach, skateboarding, and mountain biking with friends—instead of studying.

I had been banking on a strong MCAT score to overcompensate for my average-for-pre-med GPA. A competitive MCAT score is any score over 30, with 35 being considered *very* strong. In the absence of a strong GPA or some other compelling aspect of an application (like a student who worked in a lab that *actually* cured cancer), a score below 30 typically meant that the student should retake the exam and try for a higher score.

My score was a 24, well below the magic 30. Not only was I disappointed, but this also created a problem. Twenty-four was on the lower end of scores that medical schools accepted, and that was usually for students with extenuating circumstances or those who had otherwise spectacular applications. I had neither. I had been banking on a high, or at least decent, score. My insides burned with shame. I was furious with myself for not studying harder. Maybe my parents had been right to be skeptical of my prospects. Worse yet, perhaps all of the unspoken things my childhood friends' parents had indicated through their actions were true after all. Perhaps I was not cut out to succeed. The more I felt like I didn't deserve to succeed, the less I expected to. I began to lose motivation.

Of course, my adviser recommended that I re-study, take the MCAT again, and try for a higher score. This would mean delaying my ambitions of becoming a doctor by at least a year. I weighed my options. I could spend the entire year after college studying to re-take the MCAT and bolstering my extracurriculars, or I could apply right away—despite my subpar score—and hope for the best. Three years earlier, I hadn't cared about college; now I wanted more than anything to go to med school. I had to find a way. I decided to take my chances with the 24.

After I'd sent out numerous applications, weeks passed before I heard anything. Then, letters of rejection began to roll in. They all began with the classic and heartbreaking phrase, "We regret to inform you ..." By the holidays of my senior year of college, I had begun to construct a back-up plan while I prepared to retake the MCAT. Each passing week brought new letters of rejection, and I began to feel dejected. Maybe my mom had been right. Maybe I wasn't cut out for medical school. Imposter syndrome began to edge its way back into my mind like an unnoticed water leak, slowly causing damage—at first, unnoticeable, but eventually irreversible. I had believed that getting into med school would be the antidote to my deep shame, that it would forever put my feeling of inadequacy to rest. If I didn't get into med school, then what?

By January, I had finished formulating my back-up plan. It seemed like a waste of time to take an entire year off to re-apply to medical school. It was also a risk. I worried that I would lose focus, become distracted, and worst of all, find excuses not to re-apply. My solution was to leave the United States and go to medical school in the Caribbean.

Foreign medical schools admit new classes of students multiple times each year. This meant that, once I got all the painful rejections from US med schools out of the way, I could immediately apply to a fresh batch of Caribbean schools. I would apply during the spring of my senior year, interview during the summer, get accepted in the fall, and begin my first year of medical school in the winter. That would only put me six months behind my original schedule. Because the majority of Caribbean med schools are for-profit, they are motivated to fill all of the seats in their classrooms. I interpreted this to mean that they might be willing to admit someone like me, even with a lower than typical MCAT score. With this back-up plan in place, I began to feel at ease.

By pursuing med school in the Caribbean, I would be taking a huge gamble on my future self. But I was on a mission. I was desperate to prove everyone wrong: my parents, my friends' parents, all those med schools who had "regretted to inform" me. I could do this. I could go to med school. They would all have to call me doctor one day. Like a child excitedly opening birthday presents, I cast my reservations aside like old wrapping paper.

In late January, before I had a chance to begin sending out my pleas—I mean applications—to the Caribbean schools, I received an email that changed everything. I couldn't believe my eyes. "We are pleased to inform you …" appeared on my iPhone screen. A med school in Kansas City, Missouri, had invited me to interview. I must have read that email forty-five times, just to be sure. Whether intentionally or by accident, my application had somehow made its way out of the school's "no way" pile, and into the "let's consider this kid" pile. This was my shot! A gigantic grin spread across my face as I realized I *actually* had a shot! Now, all I had to do was make it through the interview.

Ring. Ring. Ring. I tapped my leg as I waited for my mom to answer her phone. I replayed in my mind that first time I had told her I wanted to go to med school, along with every conversation I'd had with her about med school since then. Each one had been less optimistic than the one before it.

Finally, she picked up. "Hello?" she said.

"You're not going to believe this!" I nearly shouted, as I struggled to contain my excitement.

"What, what is it? Are you O.K.?"

"Have you ever been to Kansas City?"

"No, I don't think so." Puzzled, she continued, "What's going on?"

"Oh, nothing much … I was just calling to see if you could help me figure out what to wear in Kansas City this time of year."

"I don't understand …"

Then, like a crowd waiting outside of Walmart as it opens its doors on the morning of Black Friday, charged with anticipation and no longer able

17

to hold back, the excitement I had been working so hard to stifle surged through into my voice, "I GOT AN INTERVIEW IN KANSAS CITY!"

A short pause, then, "Ryan, that is fantastic news!" I knew that she was grinning too, and this made me smile even bigger.

After we had both regained our composure, she said, "A suit."

"What? What do you mean?" My excitement had left me confused and a little disoriented.

"You should wear a suit."

That weekend, she took me to buy a suit for the interview. While the salesman at Men's Warehouse took my measurements, he made small talk and asked what the occasion was. Before I could answer, my mom proudly blurted out that it was for a med school interview. Even though I had overheard her telling other people, I was still not used to hearing it. Since only one med school had invited me to interview, I was still concerned that a mix-up had occurred. I worried that when I showed up for the interview, I would encounter a flustered secretary uncomfortably shuffling through papers looking for my name on the interview list, mumbling to themself that a mistake had been made, making muffled phone calls, and then apologizing for the error. Or what if they had invited the wrong Ryan McPherson?

I flew to Kansas City in February on Super Bowl Sunday and interviewed the next day. As I stepped off the plane that evening, the cold air cut through my pullover sweatshirt, like a thousand needles. It had been snowing all weekend, and factoring in the wind chill, the temperature was in the single digits. I was a California kid; I'd never been this cold before in my life. But I didn't care. This was my shot. My *only* shot.

The next morning at 6:45 a.m., I sat alone on a bench in the lobby of my hotel, wearing my new suit. I had tied and re-tied my tie five times, until I had gotten it, so the tip of the tie just barely grazed the top of my belt. That's what a YouTube video had recommended. I was already wide awake, but I sipped from a cup of hot coffee anyway, taking extreme caution not to spill any on myself. The routine brought me comfort, and besides, it was still freezing outside. The roads had been plowed and piles of snow lined the streets and driveways. In my head, I silently reviewed the interview questions I thought might be asked and how I planned to respond to each one.

I checked my watch. It was now 7:04. My ride, a shuttle provided by the medical school, was supposed to have picked me up at seven a.m. My heart began to race. I looked around the lobby hoping that I would see someone else wearing a suit like me, also waiting for the shuttle. But except for the receptionist, who was quietly shuffling papers, I was alone. My mind began to race. Had I gotten the date wrong? Had they forgotten me? Had they had realized they had only invited me by mistake and recalled the shuttle from picking me up? My heart pounded.

I stood up and began to pace around the silent lobby. The receptionist looked up and smiled courteously at me. I imagined to myself that she was wondering what I was doing there, who I was waiting for, if they had abandoned me. Maybe she was in on it! Perhaps the medical school had called and told her they weren't coming for me, that they had already decided I wasn't worth their time. Suddenly, her courteous smile felt like a smile of pity.

I continued pacing around. I checked my watch again, 7:10 a.m. The lobby felt uncomfortably warm. Sweat began to moisten my lower back. I was thinking about stepping outside for some fresh air when I became aware of a new sound, an idling engine. I spun around and faced the sliding glass lobby doors, and to my relief, I saw that a van had pulled up. I squinted so that I could see into it and noticed it was full of other people who were all dressed just like me! I nearly ran outside, fearful they would leave as quickly as they had appeared.

The driver had climbed out and opened the side door for me to get in and join everyone else. He apologized for being late, citing the weather and saying that I was the last stop. Then once I had found my seat and fastened my seatbelt, he assured us all that we wouldn't be late to the interview, our next stop.

It was about a fifteen-minute ride from the hotel to the campus. I had been expecting a quiet ride, that everyone would be as nervous as I was. I was wrong. Everyone chatted animatedly about the Super Bowl, the weather, where they had come from, and what they had heard about this med school through the pre-med grapevine.

We pulled up to the school and parked. The campus was composed of several four-story red brick buildings spread out around a courtyard, with a large brick smokestack towering over all of the other buildings. Covered in fresh snow, the scene was picturesque. I stood in awe. These buildings had been built nearly 100 years ago, and every year since, they had served as domiciles for medical students, one of which I was eager to become. The beauty and sophistication of what lay before me intimidated me and only made me more nervous. I briefly wished the campus had been hideous and covered in mud instead.

We followed the shuttle driver into the lobby of one of the buildings, where we were greeted with tables that had been laid out with coffee, pastries, and name tags. We all huddled around, pouring coffee, and searching for our name tag. I scanned the table and was relieved to see "Ryan McPherson" written in bold black letters across a white tag. I picked it up as if it was a fragile piece of jewelry and clipped it to the lapel of my suit jacket. Wearing the name tag, I felt validated, that no mistake had been made, that I *actually* belonged.

We stood around slurping on cups of hot coffee, shiny name tags dangling from our lapels. The van driver disappeared and a representative from the school took over as our new host. She outlined our agenda for the day. Throughout the morning, we would be pulled away individually for interviews with the faculty. She handed out a paper schedule that listed each of our names and the faculty members who would interview us. After we were through with the interviews, we would go on a group tour of the school to conclude the day. As soon as she had finished, the small talk from the van ride resumed.

I nibbled on a cold danish to give me something to do with my hands. I tried to look comfortable wearing my new suit, as though I had gone on plenty of interviews like this before. The small talk slowly turned from friendly banter to posturing—where else they'd interviewed, their MCAT scores, and extracurriculars that would look good on a med school application.

Students began to get called away for their individual interviews. Four or five students were pulled away before one of the secretaries came to get me for my interview. I was feeling a little bit inadequate after listening to the other interviewees' conquests of medical school interviews for the past hour.

Ok, I told myself as I followed her down a long hallway, *this is it. Nothing that happened out there matters, only what happens now.*

We stopped at a door that had been left ajar and she knocked gently.

"Come in!" came a booming male voice on the other side.

The secretary smiled at me and without saying anything gestured for me to enter before she turned and walked away. I took a deep breath and stepped inside.

It turned out the room wasn't an office after all, but instead a small conference room. A large wooden oval table sat in the middle of the room surrounded by chairs. On the far side of the table were two older men wearing suits. One was wearing glasses and had a manicured white beard. I don't remember what the other looked like. In front of them were stacks of papers. I noticed that the papers had pictures of us on them with our names printed underneath. The gentleman with the facial hair smiled, stood up, and extended his hand for me to shake. He introduced himself as Dr. Murphy.

We exchanged brief pleasantries as I sat down across from them. The last thing I wanted to think about was the person who interviewed before me, but the warmth of the seat was a forced reminder that someone else just like me had been sitting here in front of them only moments ago. My mind began to race with thoughts about how much more qualified they must be. I forced these thoughts out of my mind and focused on the two doctors in front of me.

Just that morning in the hotel lobby I had been preparing answers to potential interview questions like, "Why pick me? Why do I want to go into medicine?" stuff like that. They may have asked me those questions, but I don't remember. The interview felt like it was moving very quickly. But the one thing I do remember:

"So, you like to read?" Dr. Murphy asked, looking up from a paper that was probably my resume.

"Yes," I replied.

"What was the last book you read?" he asked, looking directly at me. Maybe he was genuinely curious or maybe he didn't believe me that reading was actually a hobby of mine. (I had left skateboarding and surfing off of the list, because they didn't seem very doctor-ly.)

My mind suddenly went blank. This was not one of the questions I had anticipated. When I finally remembered the most recent book I had read, I became nervous, afraid that this might be the wrong venue to discuss the title. But I said it anyway. *"Thank You for Smoking.* By Christopher Buckley."

There was a pause, and then Dr. Murphy chuckled, "I've read that one too, it's hilarious!"

We bantered for a bit, and then we were standing and shaking hands, and suddenly I was back in the reception area with all of the other interviewees, listening to them ask each other where they were from.

A couple of weeks later, I was sitting in my microbiology lab course listening to the professor explain the experiment we were about to conduct. I was in my final semester of college, and while I should have been celebrating my upcoming graduation, I was not. I still had no definite plan after graduating.

The professor went on, "The bacteria I am about to hand out have been growing in agar since earlier this week ..." My phone vibrated in my pocket. I silently pulled out my iPhone and glanced at it. I had a new email. An email from Kansas City. The only medical school I had interviewed at.

My heart began pounding in my chest and my palms began to sweat. This was it. Should I open it now or wait? If it began with the words "We regret to inform you ..." then I would be upset for the rest of class and people would ask me what was wrong. The last thing I wanted to do was tell them that my medical career was ending before it had even started.

My hands made the decision without my brain. I opened the email. My vision became blurry. There were a lot of words all over the screen. My heart was racing. I quickly scanned the page for the phrase "We regret to inform you ..." but I couldn't find it. I forced my brain to focus, and I started reading from the beginning, mouthing the words as I did. "Dear Ryan McPherson ..." I continued on, and as I did, the blood drained from my face, and I felt faint. Over and over again, I mouthed the next word to myself, just to be sure: "*Congratulations.*"

By now my heart was racing at a pace that was probably dangerous. Before I knew it, I was standing up, pumping my hands in the air.

"You will have to identify the bacteria ..." The professor paused and looked at me. "What's going on?" His voice disrupted my euphoria and dropped me back to Earth. The entire class stared at me.

I cleared my throat, and then carefully, scared my voice would be shaky, I somehow got out, "Err, sorry ... I just found out I got into medical school."

"Congratulations. That's great news. Terrific. Now if you don't mind, I'm going to finish explaining today's lab so that we can all get done at a decent time."

"Of course, of course. I'm just going to use the restroom real quick." I went out into the hallway and called my mom. She shared my excitement as well, maybe even more so.

Even after I'd responded to Kansas City and confirmed that I would attend, I was still paranoid that there had been a mistake. That the email had been meant for someone else and sent to me by mistake. Or maybe two Ryan McPhersons had interviewed. I had worked hard to get into medical school, yet I still believed that I could have worked even harder. My subpar MCAT score lingered in my mind, like a heavy weight. Even if they hadn't made a mistake in sending me the email, had they made a mistake in accepting me? Had they miscalculated my ability? After all, I had only been offered an interview at one medical school. What if they were wrong and all of the others who had rejected me—just like my friends' parents in childhood— were right about me, that I wasn't cut out for the rigors that lay ahead? I felt like I was wearing the clothes of a man who had been accepted to med school, but somehow, I wasn't supposed to be. Doubts like these built up in my mind, unable to clear, like dirty dishwater building up behind a clogged drain.

CHAPTER 3—My Friend Anthony

Medicine has been an adventure, one that began for me even before I got into med school. I've met interesting people every step of the way. Anthony was one of them. At first, I found him boring and sometimes repulsive. But, overall, he was a genuine-hearted person, and after we spent enough time together, like a fungus, he grew on me.

When I was a sophomore in college, I met Anthony through friends. He was two years older than I was, and six inches shorter. By exerting as little physical effort as possible, and by indulging himself in as many earthly pleasures as he could, he meticulously maintained a perfectly round figure, like a bowling ball. He would stay up late, eat fast food, and then sleep until noon the next day, regardless of whether or not he had classes. One afternoon, I discovered him asleep in his bed, covered in candy wrappers. He was the exact opposite of me. He also had a job, and I didn't.

When our friend group hung out, it wasn't uncommon for Anthony to have to leave at inopportune times "for work." This happened regardless of what we were doing, the time of day, or the day of the week. None of us knew exactly what he did for work, just that he worked for his family. Whenever we pressed him for details, he would circumvent the question with an elusive response, until one fateful day.

"Hey, you guys," Anthony started, getting our attention. "I need one of you to help me with something tomorrow afternoon."

"With what?" our friend Paul asked warily, not wanting to volunteer himself for something unpleasant.

"Something for work."

There was silence as we all considered this. Because we didn't know what Anthony did, we couldn't know what we would be volunteering for.

Finally, Anthony broke the silence. "I'll pay you."

That was good enough for broke ass me. "I'll do it," I said, trying not to sound too eager, but wanting to reply before anyone else.

"Great. I'll pick you up tomorrow afternoon, around three. Wear a button-down shirt, a tie, and slacks."

The next afternoon, I stood outside my dorm wearing a black button-down shirt, black slacks, and a red tie I had borrowed from my roommate. It was a cloudless afternoon, and the sun was beating down on me. My body threatened to perspire from every pore. I felt uncomfortable, because I normally wore shorts and a T-shirt. I pulled my phone out of my pocket and checked the time. It was 3:03 p.m. Where was he? I told myself that if Anthony didn't pull up in the next two minutes, I was going to go back inside, change, and go play Halo instead.

Just as I had made up my mind to go back inside, a minivan I'd never seen before pulled up and stopped directly in front of me. It was an older, faded silver job with tinted back windows. The passenger side window rolled down to reveal Anthony sitting behind the steering wheel, dressed similarly to me. Either the AC in the van didn't work or his body had less fortitude than mine, because he was sweating.

"Get in," he said, as he unlocked the door.

I got in beside him, relieved to feel a cool blast of air conditioning. The tires screeched as we sped off, and the campus faded away in the rear-view mirror.

For the first ten minutes, our conversation was casual. But with each passing moment, curiosity gnawed away at me.

"So," I asked, trying to sound nonchalant, "where are we going?"

"Across town," he responded immediately without taking his eyes off the road. This didn't help me much since Los Angeles is a giant place and "across town" could be anywhere. I began to grow frustrated. His evasiveness about his job was cute, bordering on annoying, when we were all just hanging out. Now that I had been enlisted to help him, I deserved to know what I had gotten myself into.

We stopped at a red light and Anthony fumbled with the radio, changing stations. I stuck my hand out and turned the radio off.

"Dude!" I said assertively. "Joke's over, you need to tell me what we are doing."

He turned and faced me, the light still red, and in a serious tone said, "We are going to move a dead body." Then the light turned green, he turned back to road, the tires screeched again, and we sped off, this time without music playing.

I didn't say anything. I figured that he was probably still trying to keep his little joke alive. As frustrated as I felt, I was going to find out eventually. But as we continued on in silence, my mind began to churn. The farther we went, the worse each scenario became. I thought about how Anthony was always going to work at odd hours ... how he had always been cagey about what it was he did, only ever telling us that he worked for his "family" ... scenes from Mafia movies began to run through my head. Wasn't Anthony an Italian name, too?!

Doing my best to hide the burgeoning terror in my voice, I cleared my throat and tried to speak, but no comprehensible sentence came out of my mouth. All I could think at that moment was, *What did I just get myself into?* Visions of being arrested, interrogated in a dingy room by a good cop and a bad cop, being tried in a court, the judge screaming at me that I would never be allowed to go to medical school ... all began zooming through my mind.

Seeing me squirm, Anthony burst out laughing, "You should have seen your face! You turned as pale as the body we are going to pick up!"

I was now thoroughly convinced that we were actually going to pick up a dead body. I wondered if now I "knew too much," and it was too late for me to bail. Would I be the next body if I did?

Trying to sound nonchalant, I finally stammered out, "That's funny, dude, but what are we *actually* doing?"

"I'm serious ... we are picking up a dead body and moving it to the mortuary."

"Mortuary?"

"Yeah, dude, I work for my parents. They own a couple of mortuaries around town, and we have to drive out to where the person died and pick them up." He motioned with his free hand to the back of the minivan, "then drop them off at the mortuary so they can be prepared for their funeral."

I looked into the back of the minivan and noticed for the first time that it had been modified. The seats had been removed and replaced by a metal stretcher that could be secured to and detached from the floor.

"I thought that's what a hearse was for?" I half-asked.

"No, those are more formal, for the actual funeral," he replied.

"Why'd we have to dress up then?"

"Unless we're picking the body up at a morgue or a hospital, then we have to go into the house where the patient died, and all of the family will be standing around, mourning. So, we have to look nice, you know, respectful." Then for good measure he added, "So, be on your best behavior, no joking around!"

I sat back in my seat and breathed a sigh of relief that I was not about to be implicated in a major crime. Then, suddenly concerned that I was about to see something that would haunt me for years and leave me with crippling PTSD, I blurted out, "We aren't going to a crime scene, are we?"

"No, dude! When we pick people up at their houses it's not because they were murdered! It's because they were very sick and dying and they wanted to spend their last days home and surrounded by loved ones. I think it's called hospice or something."

I relaxed a bit, still not entirely sure what was going to happen next. I had never seen a dead body before. I wondered how I would react. Would I run away, like in middle school, or would I be able to keep my cool?

We pulled into a quiet suburban neighborhood, much like the one I grew up in. The late afternoon sun shone through the tree-lined streets and spread warmly over the crunchy fallen autumn leaves. From the collection of cars parked in the driveway and along the curb, it was clear which house held the body.

"This is it," Anthony grunted as he pulled the minivan up behind the driveway, blocking it.

"You're blocking the driveway," I pointed out, trying to be helpful.

"I know. We won't be here very long. It's not a good idea to park too far away. It's poor form to wheel a dead body through a neighborhood. Trust me, it draws too much attention. Don't ask."

We got out of the minivan, and I followed him up the front path toward the open front door. Through the screen door, I could see the living room full of older adults all dressed in suits. They were talking in hushed voices.

Anthony opened the screen door quietly and gently knocked on the wooden door frame. A man looked up and made his way over to us. As he got closer, I could tell from his puffy eyes that he had been crying.

Anthony introduced both of us and explained why we were there. The man shook our hands, thanked us, and invited us inside. We tried to remain invisible as we followed him across the living room, through a maze of mourners. I kept my head low, so as not to disturb anyone. Despite our best efforts, I sensed the others knew why we were there. I felt like a car driving through a flock of birds.

We rounded a corner and entered a dimly lit bedroom. As my eyes adjusted, I noticed that the room had been modified. The bed had been replaced with a hospital bed and the space around it filled with numerous medical devices: IV poles, monitors, a wheelchair, bedside commode, a bedside table with several pill bottles carefully lined up. The blend of bedroom and hospital room made me feel queasy.

I braced myself. I glanced around the room, trying to avoid looking at the hospital bed directly, where I knew the body lay. The sight of numerous medical devices made me uncomfortable. I worried that my expression would reveal my discomfort. I tried to think about something else, but no matter how hard I tried, my imagination ran wild imagining what the dead body would look like.

Anthony and the man, who had revealed himself as the deceased's son, stood at the side of the bed, casually signing forms that Anthony had brought with him, not unlike a FedEx driver delivering a package. They were oblivious to my nausea and apprehension. Despite the cool temperature inside the house, I suddenly felt flushed and warm. The room began to spin. I stumbled sideways, which caused Anthony and the son to stop what they were doing and turn their attention to me. Anthony's expression conveyed, *What the fuck, man! Get it together!* The son's expression remained that of someone in mourning.

Thankfully, I didn't end up fainting. My embarrassment replaced my fear of the unknown, and that was enough to revive me. My blood pressure returned to normal. I nodded, trying to look casual, at both of them, and they turned back to what they had been doing.

I finally worked up the courage to look at the hospital bed. But there was nothing for me to see; a clean white bed sheet had been placed over the body, covering him entirely.

"We will have to wheel him through the living room," I could hear Anthony saying to the man. "It's best if you can move the guests to another part of the house while we do this, so they don't have to watch." The man nodded and headed for the living room. Anthony came over to me and hissed, "Yo! Stop acting like you've never seen a dead body before!"

"I never *have* seen a dead body before!"

"Well, it's time to pretend like you have!" he retorted.

He glared at me, and I followed him through the house back to the minivan.

Standing behind the minivan Anthony seemed to forget that he was annoyed with me. He said, "Always have them clear out. The worst thing that can happen is, you're wheeling them through a crowded room, and something happens."

"Something like what? They come back alive?!" I asked, my mind racing.

"No! Worst case scenario," he continued seriously, "you drop them in front of everyone." He paused, and then seeing the doubtful look on my face, continued, "It could happen easier than you think. Stretcher wheel gets stuck on a piece of carpet, or can't make it up over the doorway, then BOOM!" he clapped his hands together loudly, "Next thing you know, they're on the floor. Everyone is looking at you like you're an idiot. Grandma is crying. Terrible. Just terrible." He paused again, thinking, and then repeated slowly,

"Always make the family leave when you wheel the body out."

With that, he opened up the back of the minivan and pulled out the stretcher. Together, we wheeled it back up the front path to the house and stepped into the now-empty living room, pulling the metallic gurney with us. We made our way back into the converted bedroom and brought the stretcher up next to the hospital bed.

"Here." Anthony handed me a pair of purple latex medical gloves. As soon as we had both put them on, without warning, he reached up, and in a single sweeping gesture, pulled the sheet off of the hospital bed exposing the dead body.

Lying there in front of us was an old man who looked like he was sleeping peacefully. If I hadn't been told he was dead, I might not have known. His eyes were closed, and his arms lay at his side. It felt like we would wake him up if we weren't quiet. The sight was not nearly as horrifying as I had built up in my mind.

Anthony interrupted my thoughts, explaining that we had to move him quickly before people started trickling back into the living room. "And remember, no matter what, don't drop the body!"

I nodded my understanding.

Anthony placed his hands on the man's shoulder, and I grabbed his ankles, which were cold.

"On the count of three." Anthony began to count, "One … two … three!"

We swung the man over onto our stretcher. He was so frail I was afraid we would break him, but he remained intact. I peeked at his face to see if he had opened his eyes, just in case we were removing someone who wasn't really dead. He had not, and we were not.

We re-covered the man with a white sheet, wheeled him back through the empty living room, out of the house, back down the front path, and pushed the stretcher into the back of the minivan without any difficulties. Anthony went back inside briefly to let the man's son know that we were finished and would be leaving.

Driving away I felt like I needed to say something, so I asked, "Where to now?"

"Blue Lotus Mortuary"

"Where is that?"

"Literally right across the street from campus."

I had never noticed.

A while later we pulled up to Blue Lotus and unloaded the minivan. Getting him into the mortuary was less of an ordeal than getting him out of his home. After we had finished, we got back into the van.

"I feel like having a milkshake" Anthony said, turning to me. "Do you want a milkshake?"

I did not want a milkshake, but I nodded anyway.

After a quick stop at McDonald's, Anthony dropped me back in front of my dorm, exactly where he had picked me up several hours earlier. He handed me a twenty-dollar bill. I had completely forgotten I was getting paid.

Later that week, Anthony asked me if I could help him out more often. By then, several days had passed and I had been able to reflect on the experience. I realized two things: 1) Like a child being thrown into a pool and forced to learn how to swim, I had survived my first encounter with a corpse. Until then, I hadn't thought that I'd be able to do that. And 2) This job might be a good way to help desensitize me to some of my phobias of sickness and death. After all, I did want to become a physician ... right?

For the next year, we drove all over Los Angeles County. We walked through countless fluorescent hospital basements and out through their back doors, visited homes in neighborhoods of L.A. that I had never known existed. My discomfort around dead bodies began to dissipate.

The following year, Anthony graduated and moved away. I still had another year to go. We fell out of touch, but whenever I see an old minivan, I think of Anthony, and I wonder what might be inside.

* * *

Med school turned out to be harder than I'd expected. The four years are broken into two equal parts. The first two years are taught in a lecture hall and various labs around campus, and the second two years are hands-on teaching in the hospital. During the first two years of med school, every day was similar; every morning for four hours we would attend lectures, then have lunch for an hour, then spend an additional four hours in the afternoon either in more lectures or doing a lab, then finally, we would go home and study. We had a myriad of labs to attend; the most dreaded was cadaver lab.

In cadaver lab, we spent the year meticulously dissecting rigid, lifeless people who had donated their bodies to science. The lab was in the med school basement, just below the lecture hall. The basement was a large, brightly lit fluorescent room with tile walls, giving it the impression that the entire place could be cleaned with a hose. Spread throughout the room were cold metal tables. Lying on each table was a sealed black body bag. Within each bag lay the body of a human being, recently deceased and preserved with various chemicals. More striking than the sight of corpses was the penetrating aroma of formaldehyde and other caustic smells.

On the first day of cadaver lab, we were randomly assigned to groups of five students. Each group was then assigned a cadaver. We were to unzip the body bags and meet our cadaver for the year, for the first time. There was a restless, nervous chatter throughout the lab. When it finally came time to open the zippered black bags, there was a cacophony of zippers being unzipped, followed by silence. *Dead* silence. The sight of a dead body was a shock to most, and everyone did their best to maintain their composure. As I looked around the room, I appreciated the range of different body types included in the cadaver population: tall, fat, short, skinny, male, female, Black, white, Hispanic, Asian, old, youngish (though no children, thankfully). It was as if everyone waiting in line at the supermarket one afternoon had suddenly died and had been taken here.

I glanced around the cold room. There was a mixture of expressions ranging from people with frowns, to those with eyes closed, to others gritting their teeth. One student had to step out into the hall, where she collapsed. Shockingly, the sight of dead bodies before me did not disturb me one bit. Which is surprising, because nearly every bodily function of a still-alive

32

person still did.

Despite my experiences with Anthony, I hated every second of cadaver lab. Several afternoons every week, for hours, we would stand and watch our anatomy professor meticulously skin and dissect his cadaver, uncovering, identifying, and naming subtle anatomic structures just beneath the skin: nerves, arteries, veins, ligaments, tendons, muscles, and bones. Then, we would regroup around our assigned cadavers and attempt to replicate his handiwork. We did this for weeks, until our cadavers all looked like they were on loan from *Bodies: The Exhibition*.

I found dissecting to be tedious, and the endless naming of various little, squishy, dead, parts of the human body boring. I did not get excited like other students did when they uncovered an anatomic variance. Unlike physiology, which required contemplation, anatomy consisted of brute memorization. By the time our first anatomy test was scheduled, I estimated that we'd memorized at least 1,000 structures in the human body. I'd never taken an anatomy class before and learning this many new Latin vocabulary words felt like trying to drink from a firehose.

For the exam, the cadavers had been arranged so that they lined the walls of the anatomy lab in a circular fashion. They had then been covered with drapes exposing just a small area of dissection. Within this small area, a tiny pin with a number on its end had been placed. Students were then brought into the room in groups and placed individually in front of a numbered pin. For sixty seconds we were allowed to examine (without touching) the exposed (and often unrecognizable) area of dissection, and then write down the name of the structure in which the pin had been placed. Then a bell would sound, and everyone would silently move sideways to the next station. This continued until we had examined all fifty pins.

We received our exam results a few days later, just before our first holiday break. I had failed. My heart sank. My med school career was again in jeopardy. For the first time in years, I cried. The voice telling me I was an imposter and that I'd never amount to anything, much less become a doctor, came back with a vengeance.

As it turned out, I wasn't alone. A substantial portion of my class had also failed the exam. Instead of kicking us all out, the anatomy department hosted a one-time make-up exam, scheduled for one week later—during our first holiday break. I seized the opportunity and cancelled my travel arrangements to visit my family in California. Instead, I spent all day, every day, in the anatomy lab, diligently studying each cadaver. In the evenings, I ran through flash cards and devoured anatomy textbooks. Growing up, I had rarely played team sports, and this was the first time I felt truly under pressure to perform.

At the end of that week, I stood in the anatomy lab and faced the cadavers which had been rearranged around the room and covered, just as before. I bent over, examined the pin in front of me, and then scribbled down my answer. The bell sounded and I stepped to my left and began again.

That afternoon, I sat nervously in my apartment, unsure if I should celebrate or start packing my bags. My phone buzzed, alerting me to a new email from the school. The email was to inform us that the exams had been graded and posted online. I took a deep breath and logged in on my MacBook. There was a long pause as the webpage struggled to load. As it did, my eyes frantically raced around the screen searching for my new test score. And then, I found it: "Pass." Hallelujah! I was still in the game. Relief like I had never experienced before washed over me, drowning me in euphoria. "That was a close call," I thought. "Good thing I don't want to become a surgeon."

After surviving anatomy, I felt renewed. But med school didn't become any less of a challenge. The lectures and information continued to come at speeds that left me dizzy. As the year went on, our class was ranked based on our grades. The top 10% of the class earned the faux-derogatory term "gunner," bestowed upon them by the bottom 90% of the class. My friends and I would teasingly accuse each other of "gunning" whenever we discovered one another studying more than the rest. Although it was a joke on the surface, we all secretly wanted to be gunners. Every single person in the class did.

One spring afternoon toward the end of my first year of med school, I was walking back to my apartment. I felt particularly overwhelmed and discouraged after a series of especially brutal lectures. Then I overheard a group of second year students talking as they walked in front of me.

"Med school is easy," one of them said to another.

What a pompous ass, I thought to myself.

"You really think so?" the other student asked.

"Yeah, I do. You only have to do two things."

This captured my attention. I sped up, not wanting to miss what was next. Maybe he would offer a critical piece of secret advice that could help propel me to *gunner*-hood.

"Oh yeah, and what would those two things be?" his friend asked.

"Put your head down, and study!" the first one said, and they both burst out laughing.

Initially I was disappointed to find out that he was telling a joke instead of doling out legitimately helpful advice. But his words ran through my mind for the rest of the afternoon, "Med school is easy. All you have to do is put your head down and study." Even though he was joking, he was still on to something. Despite the joke, I found his simplification of med school helpful. For the remainder of my four years as a medical student, whenever I found myself feeling overwhelmed, I repeated these words to myself, and they helped me calm down and refocus.

In the spring of the second year of med school, all med students in the entire country have to take a national standardized exam called the *USMLE Step 1*, or Step 1, for short. Forty-five very long days after taking the exam, each student receives a three-digit score. This score determines which medical or surgical specialties a student will or will not be able to pursue after graduating medical school. For example, specialties like dermatology and neurosurgery are considered "highly competitive" and generally require graduating at the top of one's class from a top medical school, as well as a very high Step 1 score. I had no idea what type of doctor I wanted to become but I—at the very least—didn't want to close any doors by doing poorly on the exam. Because of my near-miss with the MCAT, I did not take preparing for Step 1 lightly. "Just put your head down and study," I kept telling myself.

I took the test in June and then retreated back to California to spend a few carefree weeks of my summer break with friends and family. I tried not to think about the test, but I couldn't push it out of my mind.

At the end of July, I returned to pack up my apartment. I was moving closer to the hospital where I would spend the third and fourth years of medical school. As I was driving on the freeway toward my new apartment, my phone buzzed in my pocket.

I pulled off the road, closed my eyes, took a deep breath, and mentally prepared for both the best—and the worst—case scenarios. Just like in microbiology lab two years earlier, with my heart racing, I opened the email. As cars whizzed by, I scanned my iPhone's screen until my eyes landed on three bolded numbers: **239**. This score was well above average. Not only was it above average, it was high enough to differentiate me from my peers when it came time to apply for residency. My efforts had paid off. I pulled my car back onto the freeway and smiled. For the first time, I felt I had been crazy to have ever thought the school had made a mistake by inviting me to come interview two years ago on that cold February day.

CHAPTER 4—Code Grey

N ow that I had survived the first two years of med school, it was time to leave the classroom behind and start learning on the job. For the final two years of med school, I'd be in the hospital, working among physicians, residents, nurses, and patients. *Actual* patients. Years three and four are known collectively as "clinical rotations." These are designed to give us exposure to different medical specialties, so we can discover what type of medical specialty we want to practice. Every month we would rotate between core specialties like family medicine, internal medicine, general surgery, psychiatry, pediatrics, intensive care, emergency medicine, and obstetrics and gynecology. After completing these, we were then allowed to select other non-core specialties we were interested in, such as orthopedic surgery, radiology, anesthesiology, rheumatology, to name a few.

Although we had all made it through the first two years of medical school and had *technically* been taught "medicine," as I stepped into the hospital, it felt like I was starting all over again, just like J.D. Here, no one cared if you knew how many ATP molecules were generated at the end of the Krebs cycle, or which enzyme in the brain was responsible for making dopamine. In the real world, the skills we needed to acquire were things like how to take a thorough history and perform a physical exam, interpret laboratory and imaging results, and then keep track of all of these data points. This was even more complex than it sounds, because the data points changed daily for all of the patients. At times, I felt like a supercomputer. A very tired supercomputer.

Eventually, once I had started to acclimate, the process began to feel routine: patient comes to the hospital complaining of X, I ask patient several questions about X and then examine them head to toe, review patient's labs, look at patient's imaging, attempt to determine what is wrong with patient, select an appropriate way to treat patient. Then I'd go proudly report all of this to the supervising resident, who—if they had time—*might* listen. I quickly came to realize that my existence in the hospital didn't matter. It was all for practice. The final decisions were made by the residents and the attending physicians. My job was to try to absorb their thought processes and hone my critical thinking skills.

When I worked in the hospital, it was not uncommon for my days to be disrupted by various emergencies. These typically came in the form of "codes." Just like in the movies, the "code" would be announced overhead, for example, "Code blue to room 662!" Codes are ways of urgently alerting medical staff and doctors to an emergency. The most famous "code" is a "code blue." Code blue refers to cardiac arrest, or more simply put, a patient's heart stopping beating, meaning that they had literally just died.

Once a code blue is called, it becomes a race against time to try to revive the patient. Moments after the code blue is announced overhead, an army of nurses, doctors, and various other hospital staff descend on the patient like vultures onto roadkill, all charged with adrenaline, and eager to help. Each person in the room has a designated job to perform, and it becomes the duty of the physician—who stands at the foot of the bed—to supervise and lead their army's campaign against death.

As med students, we were often assigned the role of performing chest compressions. We would line up along the patient's left side, and every two minutes, we'd take turns pushing downward onto the patient's chest 120 times per minute in an attempt to circulate the patient's blood and keep their brain alive. The first person to push on the patient's chest usually had the cringeworthy experience of hearing several loud crunches and feeling the patient's ribs and breastbone breaking underneath their hands. After a few rounds of chest compressions, we would be out of breath and glistening.

Just like in the movies, sometimes code blues ended with a doctor shouting "CLEAR!" and then shocking the patient with the defibrillator. Unlike in the movies, however, this rarely led to the patient being revived.

A code blue is not the only code. Code blue is standardized among all hospitals; the other codes are not; they vary from hospital to hospital. I learned this lesson when I went to a *code grey*.

Just after lunch one afternoon, I heard a "code grey" announced overhead, and was curious. I had just begun third year and had caught on to the fact that "codes" meant action. I raced upstairs.

When I got to the patient's room, I did a double take to make sure I was in the right place. The usual scene of bedlam was absent. Instead, there were two hospital security guards casually milling around outside the patient's room, chatting. As I approached, I could hear voices just inside the doorway, but again, I noticed that the typical commotion was absent.

"Is this the code gray?" I asked one of the security guards.

"It is," he replied as his eyes searched the front of my chest for my ID badge.

I walked into the room and found four people inside: the patient—a short, balding man in his late sixties, his nurse, and two more security guards. The patient was sitting on the edge of his bed wearing a hospital gown that kept falling forward off of his shoulders. While he talked, he kept reaching up to pull it back on.

"I need to go to work, goddamnit!" he said, raising his voice.

"You're in the hospital," his nurse replied, somewhat bored. I gathered that she had been having this conversation with him for a while now.

He tried to stand up, but the security guards stepped forward, each of them grasped one of his arms, and gently made him sit back down. This back and forth continued, and with each exchange the patient became more and more agitated.

"I need to go to work! I'm late! My supervisor is waiting for me, the phone lines won't lay themselves!" Now he was yelling and swiping away the security guards' hands each time they tried to compel him to sit back down.

I had never seen a disoriented patient before, and I was intrigued. Everyone

39

around me seemed bored by the scene, like it was routine, but I was new, and this was new to me. How would it end?

Soon the patient's frustration reached a head and he started acting more aggressively, swinging at the security guards with closed fists. Against their resistance, he managed to stand up, and as he shook himself free of them, his gown slid off of his shoulders, falling completely off into a crumpled pile on the floor. He didn't even notice. As he stood there, naked, he continued to try fight off the security guards, the entire time shouting about how he was late for work.

Transfixed by the patient, I hadn't noticed that a second nurse had slipped into the room, carrying with her a needle and a syringe. The security guards glanced at her, and she nodded. Suddenly, they grabbed his arms and in one swift movement, pinned him down on the bed while the nurse pushed the needle into his shoulder, administering some sort of tranquilizer.

The medication worked much faster than I had anticipated. For a moment, it seemed to have no effect, other than to agitate the patient further, but then slowly, I could see him becoming weaker and weaker, as if he was rapidly falling asleep. After two minutes the same guards he had been fighting were helping him climb underneath the covers.

Back in bed he sat up, still naked, and began to cry, helplessly, "I just want to go to work ... I've worked for the telephone company for thirty-five years, just let me go ..."

His voice trailed off and eventually he lay back in bed, limp and asleep. His nurse tended to him, and the guards turned and left leaving me silently standing there, feeling awkward, as if I had seen something that I was not supposed to see.

In the elevator, I stared at the floor, thinking about what I had just seen. It had not been what I had expected, a thrilling *code blue* in which split-second decisions were used to save someone's life. Instead, it had been replaced with the sad scene of a confused and dying man.

When I got back downstairs, I dug around in my backpack and found the sheet of laminated paper the hospital had given us on our first day with the list of codes and what they were. There it was, in the middle of the list, "*code gray* ... agitated patient."

Later, I asked one of the internal medicine residents about what had happened. He told me that medical personnel usually don't respond to code grays, just security. I asked him about the injection the nurse had given the patient. He told me that it was probably a "B-52," a potent combination of the three tranquilizing medications: lorazepam, haloperidol, and Benadryl.

"By the way," he asked me, "which patient was it?"

"Room 332," I replied.

"Ahh," he said knowingly, "Mr. Genfield."

He gave me a sideways glance to see my reaction and by the expression on my face he could tell that he had succeeded in holding me in suspense, like a kid dying to know what happened next on their favorite cartoon.

"Mr. Genfield has metastatic prostate cancer. Some of it has metastasized to his brain, which is why he gets confused from time to time."

Reading my mind, he continued.

"Unfortunately, it's so advanced that there is not much more that can be done other than keep him comfortable and safe from accidentally hurting himself."

His pager beeped and he pulled it off of his waistband, looked at it, made a sour face and without a word, he walked away.

In the hospital, a lot of unsettling things happen. Patients will vomit, bleed, pee, poop, cough, yell, scream, cry, and spit. Blood pours out of every orifice. Feet die and toes fall off. Eyeballs get punctured. Brains spill out of heads ... and more. Meanwhile, unique and pungent smells accompany this brew of human bodily fluids. And sometimes, patients die. After pointing this out to me, a radiologist, who generally works away from patients, once asked me, "Are you sure you want to work in a hospital?"

For some reason, I was.

CHAPTER 5—Definitely Not Surgery

My first clinical rotation of third year—my first year in the hospital—was general surgery. The one specialty I had decided early on that I *definitely* did not want to do.

My failure in anatomy lab aside, surgeons have the reputation of being arrogant jocks. On top of that, I had heard numerous stories of med students passing out in the O.R. during surgery. Although I was comfortable around dead bodies—*thanks, Anthony*—I was still somewhat queasy around blood. I wanted nothing to do with surgery. But it was required, so I had to do it.

Every morning of that month, I got to the hospital at five a.m. and chased the surgical team around the hospital until the evening and sometimes late into the night. In the early morning, we would do "rounds" and see our post-operative patients in their rooms. We'd wake them up and ask them the same three questions as fast as possible: "How's your pain?" "Have you eaten anything?" and most importantly, "Have you had a bowel movement?"

After this, we'd race down to the operating room to begin our first *case* (surgery) at seven-thirty a.m. In between cases, while the operating room was being *turned over* (cleaned and prepared for the next surgery), we would race back and forth around the hospital from the operating room to the emergency room to see new consults. Sometimes these were people with run-of-the-mill appendicitis; other times, we saw people who had been brought in as *traumas* after being shot or stabbed. From there, we would then run back and forth between the emergency room and patient wards, getting back to the operating room just in time to begin the next case. There was always something going on, something new to see, something to do, and more to learn. Aside from the constant hustle, what I admired most about surgeons is that they always seemed to know what to do. Whenever another medical specialty became stumped about a patient's condition, or the patient suddenly became more ill, they would consult surgery, and we—I was proud to be a part of the team, even though I wasn't really a contributing member—would offer potentially lifesaving recommendations, usually in the form of a surgical procedure. It became easy to understand why surgeons might be misconstrued as arrogant.

My first time in the operating room, I was terrified I would pass out and embarrass myself. I did not want to start off this new chapter of my medical career being known as the guy who was squeamish around blood and guts … even though I was.

I stood in the cold, bright, operating room for the first time and held my breath. In front of me was the patient, who had been purposefully rendered unrecognizable by placing sterile surgical drapes over every part of her except for her abdomen—where we would be operating. The intent was not to disguise her, but to isolate the surgical field for sterility purposes. Secretly, I was glad for this. I was afraid that if I could see her face when we made our first incision, and if she grimaced, I would faint.

In the background was the familiar beep-beep-beep of the monitors, assuring us that although the patient was asleep and not moving, she was still alive. The anesthesiologist, Dr. Landry, craned his head over the drapes, impatient for us to begin. We were there to take out this patient's gallbladder, the most common procedure performed by general surgeons. I had never seen this surgery performed before, and my curiosity was beating out my apprehension. The attending surgeon, Dr. Herald, stood on the other side of the patient. He took a long needle and plunged it horizontally into the skin of the patient's abdomen. The needle skived sideways, just barely underneath the top layers of the skin and then with the needle still buried in her flesh, Dr. Herald lifted it up, tenting the skin up around the needle in an unnatural way that I imagined would have been extremely painful had she been awake. Then he injected the anesthetic and underneath the thin layers of skin I could see the chemical pooling together, leaving behind a bubble after the needle was withdrawn.

Dr. Herald had done this casually in just two seconds, although to me, it had seemed like longer. As I watched, I felt as though I was feeling what the patient was not—the needle going into my own skin, my own skin being pulled and tented up, and the burning of the medication as it pooled in my own flesh. I grimaced and braced myself, not sure what would happen next. Then, he handed the syringe to me and told me to do the same on my side of the patient's abdomen. I took the needle from him with a trembling hand. I stared at it and appreciated its size. It looked even bigger in my hand than it had in his just a moment ago.

"C'mon, we don't have all day here," he growled impatiently.

"Yeah, before she wakes up, please!" the anesthesiologist chimed in from the top of the bed.

Before she wakes up?! Is that really going to happen?! I thought to myself, suddenly alarmed.

My arm, acting without the appropriate go-ahead from my brain, took the needle, and in one unexpectedly smooth movement plunged the needle into the patient's skin. I froze in disbelief at what I had just done. I was amazed at how easy it had been.

"Now inject some local, c'mon, let's go!" Dr. Herald's impatience felt like pressure.

Then, just like he had, I tented up the skin and injected the medication, which formed a small bubble underneath the skin. I removed the needle. I had done it. It felt strange to me to push the needle into a living human being, but I had done it. And I hadn't fainted!

"Great," Dr. Harold remarked sarcastically, unaware of how big a moment this had been for me. "Now we can finally start." He took a scalpel and plunged it into the patient's skin where he had bubbled the anesthetic, made a small incision, and then passed the scalpel across the sleeping patient's abdomen and told me to do the same. With less hesitation this time, I copied what he had done. In my mind I imagined a marching band playing in celebration of what I had just accomplished. Dr. Harold merely grunted and told me the incision could be straighter next time.

Through small steps like this, my discomfort with the human body began to dissipate. It became replaced with an unquenchable curiosity—and then a desire to find out just how much further I could go. For the rest of the month, I found it thrilling each time we took a scalpel and cut someone open, exposed their insides, and saw parts of the body that non-surgeons never get to see in a living person. We would take a patient who was on the verge of death to the operating room and use our hands and our brains to pull them back to life. It became one of the most invigorating feelings I had ever experienced. It was like a code blue, but on steroids. I was hooked. Addicted. And just like any other addiction, this one would become the prevailing force in my life, affecting every decision I made from then on.

After that first month, I found a way to turn each clinical rotation into a *surgical* rotation. For example, during my pediatrics rotation, if I'd been helping to care for a kid who was scheduled to go to the O.R. for a procedure, I would find a way to go too, even if it meant staying late. I would find the surgeon ahead of time and ask if I could assist. Thrilled that someone was interested in what they were doing, they always said yes. Not only was this an opportunity to feed my new addiction and learn about new surgeries, but also it was a chance to impress the attending surgeons with my ever-expanding fund of surgical knowledge. In my free time, I would read surgical textbooks, practice tying knots, and hang out in the O.R. between cases to learn the names of all of the surgical instruments. In the O.R., I stood out among my peers, and when rounding on surgical patients with the team, I was a stud. Finally, I was a "gunner," a title I wore proudly.

I kept this up for the entire year, and the attending surgeons grew accustomed to my presence. By this point, it was no secret that I wanted to become a surgeon. In order to do so, though, I needed their letters of recommendation for surgical residency. To get these recommendations, I had to continue to put in the work and stand out from my peers. It didn't matter what rotation I was on, or what my other responsibilities were. Impressing surgeons was my top priority. This became problematic, as when other clinical rotations became busy and pulled me away from the O.R. I became worried that if I wasn't around as much as before, the surgeons would forget about me, or worse, assume I had lost interest in surgery. I'd been working harder than I ever had in my life, and I was not going to let this opportunity fall through my fingers. I was determined to remain a presence in the O.R.

During one of my internal medicine rotations toward the end of third year, I got an idea. Every day at noontime, the residents and medical students were required to attend an hour-long medical lecture. This daily lecture had been arranged by Dr. Vishmar, who was in charge of medical education at the hospital. We called him Dr. V. He was an internal medicine physician who no longer practiced, and he was not a huge fan of surgery. I thought maybe he'd had a bad experience on a surgical rotation when he was a med student, or maybe he believed the myth that all surgeons were arrogant. Every day, just before noon, all the students in the hospital would politely excuse themselves from whatever they were doing so that they could attend lecture. This wasn't very disruptive to hospital operations, except in the O.R., where this sudden purge of students was particularly noticeable. The surgeons usually made the students feel like crap on a shoe for leaving the O.R., even for a mandatory lecture.

I decided that this was my opportunity. I was not going to go to the lecture. I was going to stay in the O.R.

I stood in the operating room holding the retractor and eyeing the digital wall clock out of the corner of my eyes as the big red numbers flipped from 12:00 to 12:01. I was now officially late and would be counted as absent. A bead of sweat started to form on the back of my neck. I took a deep breath. There was no going back on my decision now. The room was quiet. The only sound was the "beep-beep-beep" of the anesthesia monitor. A few more minutes passed, and I began to wonder if I had made a mistake. Had anyone even noticed?

Then, without looking up and pretending to be only mildly interested, Dr. Jargons asked, "Don't you need to leave?"

Trying to play it cool, "Not until we are done here."

"Ohhhh!" Mary, the scrub tech, said sarcastically.

"Good man," Dr. Jargons replied, and then the room returned to silence as he focused on what he had been doing.

It wasn't much, but I knew my actions had been noticed. Underneath my surgical mask I was smiling. I felt like I belonged.

After doing this for a week, I began to receive vague warnings from some of the internal medicine residents that I would not be allowed to miss any more lectures. Since they were coming from the residents and not from Dr. V. himself, I didn't take the warnings seriously. While other medical students peeled off their surgical gowns every day at noon time, I continued to stake my place in the O.R., skipping lectures.

One afternoon the following week, I was told to report to Dr. V.'s office immediately. I entered the office and sat down. Opposite me, behind the desk were Dr. V., his secretary, and another clinical physician. They were silent and severe looking as they watched me take my seat. As I looked up at them, my stomach dropped. This was worse than getting called to the principal's office. I knew I was in trouble.

Throughout med school, I had never gotten in trouble. By this point, I saw myself as a bona fide gunner, the surgeons' pet. As I'd walked into Dr. V.'s office that afternoon, I'd been sure that I could make my case by arguing that I was an otherwise good medical student whose only shortfall what that I was just *super-interested* in surgery. I'd convinced myself that I was the good guy. But that was not how they saw it. From their perspectives, I hadn't just been missing lecture, I'd been defying their authority. In a hospital, clearly defined lines of authority and responsibility can make the difference between life and death. A hospital has to function as a well-oiled machine, or people die. Those were the stakes of my rebellion ... at least, according to Dr. V.

For the next thirty minutes Dr. V. and the other physician used a combination of increasing volume and harsh language to get their point across: that what I had been doing was unacceptable. The entire time, Dr V.'s secretary sat quietly jotting down notes. Although I was genuinely shaken, I remained calm, hoping that a harsh talking-to would be the end of it. But they weren't done yet. Dr. V. had still to drop his atomic bomb.

"Because of your capricious actions, I am going to fail you for your surgery rotation."

He had hit me right where he knew it would hurt. Devastated, my jaw fell open. I could not believe what I had just heard.

Was he joking? Not only had I worked my tail off, but I had been busting my ass all year with the goal of getting surgical letters of recommendation. Dr. V. and the other physician Dr. Stamph knew it, too. They also knew that with a surgical rotation "fail" on my transcript, no surgical residency program would ever consider me. They would never even give me the chance to explain what had happened. Would these men really jeopardize my career, just like that, over something that seemed so *petty*?

I walked out of his office in a state of shock. I called the dean of my medical school and recounted the story to him, asking for help. He told me that there was nothing he could do, that ultimately it was up to Dr. V.'s discretion. I couldn't believe what I heard. I felt as dejected as when I'd failed my first anatomy exam.

Over the next several days, my initial shock turned to anger and frustration. After about a week, my head finally began to clear. I discussed the situation with one of my friends, and I figured out what to do. Dr. V. was not failing me because he thought that my missing lectures had jeopardized my medical education. He was punishing me because I, a lowly third-year medical student, by ignoring his planned noon lecture, had defied him and made him feel disrespected. Damaging his ego had gotten me into this mess, so perhaps stroking it could get me out.

That evening, I went home and wrote a formal letter to Dr. V. I apologized and admitted my fault. I underscored how badly I wanted to become a surgeon, and I begged him for a second chance. Then I apologized more. I was still pretty upset when I wrote it, and it took me several drafts to finally remove all the defensive language. Then, I clicked send, emailing it to him.

The next day, Dr. V. called me back into his office. He was willing to negotiate. The letter had worked. He agreed not to fail me for my surgery rotation, but I still had to be punished. The terms of my punishment were as follows: 1) Under no circumstance could I miss another noontime lecture. This was an obvious one, and it really sucked because it required me to once again cancel my upcoming vacation plans to visit my family. 2) After I was done with my clinical duties for the day on Fridays, I would then have to drive to another affiliated hospital forty-five minutes away, where I would work the night shift with the emergency department residents. 3) In Dr. V.'s final public demonstration of victory over me, I had to give a presentation on professionalism at the very noontime conference that I had been skipping. It was harsh and humbling, but doable.

I later told the surgeons what had happened. Half-jokingly one of them said to me, "Just like a true surgeon! You got into trouble, but you figured out how to get out." It was a proud moment for me. My burgeoning surgical career was back on track.

In retrospect, Dr. V.'s punishment was a blessing in disguise. Sort of. I was convinced I wanted to become a surgeon, but there was still one *tiny* shred of doubt in my mind. Surgery had—and has—a reputation for being the most brutal residency to get through. Those who make it through are rewarded with one of the most lifestyle-unfriendly and stressful careers on the planet. Was it *really* worth it? Sure, I found surgery fascinating now, but would I always feel that way?

On the other hand, emergency medicine (EM) was the polar opposite of surgery. It had a reputation for being a particularly lifestyle-friendly career, because it's entirely composed of shift work. Ironically, emergency medicine is fairly predictable. Or at least, the schedule is. EM physicians always know ahead of time when they are going to work, and when they will be finished. There are no last-minute surgeries that regularly prevent them from going home. No patients that call them after hours. And they would never be called back into the hospital once they had left. No career in medicine is perfect, but on paper, this one was enticing. I embraced the opportunity to experience it for myself.

Just before midnight during my second assigned Friday night emergency medicine shift, a code blue was called overhead. I stiffened and turned toward the emergency medicine resident that I had been assigned to. We were standing in a patient's room, listening to him describe the neck pain that he had been having for almost a year. Yet tonight, he had decided to seek emergency medical attention.

Hearing the overhead page, the resident held up a finger to the patient, and this abruptly ended the patient's sentence about how narcotics were the only way to relieve his neck pain. The resident then looked up at the ceiling where the announcement was pouring out of the speakers: "CODE BLUE ROOM 302. CODE BLUE ROOM 302. CODE BLUE ROOM 302."

He turned to me, "C'mon." As we walked out of the room, he looked back over his shoulder and said to the patient, "I am not going to prescribe you narcotics for your neck pain. You will have to follow up with your primary physician." The patient sat there in a huff.

The resident turned back to me. "Don't worry about him. He comes into the ER once or twice a week asking for narcotics for some pain or another. Every time we work him up, there's nothing wrong."

"Gotcha." We walked briskly down the hall toward room 302, and other members of the code team—nurses, lab techs, and more—joined us along the way. By the time we arrived at room 302, we were a small army.

The resident pushed his way through the mass of people to reach the patient's bedside. First, he felt the patient's neck for a pulse. Finding none, he confirmed the patient was in cardiac arrest. Then, like a general leading a charge, he began directing the resuscitation. He had a quiet authority and spoke loud enough to be heard without yelling.

"Has epi been given?"

A voice from somewhere in the crowd, "Yes, at 23:04. One minute until the next dose."

"What rhythm has there been on the monitor?"

Someone else in the crowd responded, "P-E-A."

"How's our IV access?"

Another voice, "Good, we have two eighteens."

"Ok, give an amp of calcium and an amp of bicarb. Continue CPR and get ready for a pulse check in thirty seconds..."

This exchange continued for thirty minutes, as we exhausted every effort to revive the patient. I stood quietly in the corner of the room and watched. The patient who had arrested was a slender man with greying hair, in his sixties. I watched as he lay naked and lifeless on the hospital bed. His extremities flailed about like a rag doll as the team performed the violent-but-necessary chest compression, breaking his ribs and attempting to coax his heart into beating again. On his exposed abdomen was a fresh surgical dressing, which concealed the wound from a recent operation.

I looked around the room and noticed that, in addition to the usual hospital staff dressed in scrubs, on the other side of the room, in a dark corner, was an intruder, a civilian who shouldn't have been there. A woman about the same age as the patient, dressed in street clothes, wept inaudibly. She was clearly his wife. She had been there when her husband's heart stopped and was now watching our barbaric attempts to restart it. I felt ashamed that she was seeing what CPR looks like first-hand, and I wondered what she thought of the chaos.

Then, from the shadows near her, an arm reached out and placed a hand on her shoulder. I followed the arm to its source. Standing next to her was an older man in scrubs who wore a white coat, surgical cap, and a solemn expression. The surgeon rubbed the wife's shoulder gently, attempting to comfort her. I realized that he was the surgeon who had just operated on her husband.

Interrupting this scene was the emergency medicine resident's voice, "I'm going to call it unless anyone has any other ideas." It was the all too familiar punctuation to most code blues.

Silently, everyone looked around to see if anyone believed more could be done for this man. Knowing the patient's wife was watching, I wanted to speak up and offer a suggestion, but I couldn't think of one that made sense. We had been trying to resuscitate him for over thirty minutes and we had exceeded the limits of what modern medicine had to offer.

"Time of death, 23:39." The resident pulled off his latex gloves, and without saying anything further, walked out of the room and back down the hallway to the emergency department. He still had seven hours left of his shift. For him, the code had just been something that happens at work. Now that it was over, he had already moved on and was shifting his attention to the next patient who had been waiting in the emergency department for hours.

As everyone else began to shuffle out of the room, I stayed, frozen, my eyes transfixed on the patient's wife and surgeon. Aside from the four of us—the fourth being her dead husband—the room was now completely empty and silent. The surgeon, with his hand still on the wife's shoulder, led her closer to her now-deceased husband so that she could be with him. A white sheet had been pulled over his body leaving his head exposed. His eyes were closed, and he looked as if he was sleeping peacefully, just like the recently deceased that Anthony and I used to pick up. I watched as she reached underneath the sheet and grasped his lifeless hand. I felt out of place, getting a unique glimpse into the human side of medicine. Something that can't be taught in a lecture hall our read in a textbook. Neither of them paid any attention to me.

As the two of them stood at his bedside, I could see their expressions clearly in the light. As she held her husband's hand she began sobbing; she buried her face into the surgeon's chest. Now that the commotion had ended, I could hear parts of what the surgeon was saying, "... we've been dealing with this for so long, he put up of a hell of a fight, more than anyone else I've ever seen before ... I could tell he really loves you and that you being here with him through everything meant to world to him ... I'm so sorry it had to end like this ..." The expression on his face told me that he genuinely shared her pain.

Through her tears, "I know you did everything that you could, thank you so much for everything, and for being here now."

From these snippets of conversation, I realized that these three people had spent a great deal of time getting to know each other, that they had all been through hell together, fought for life together, and eventually lost. This sacred doctor-patient relationship had made the surgeon family to them. He was someone that they knew they could count on. Someone that would be there for them day or night if they needed him. Even now, late on Friday night after the doctor-patient relationship had ended and everyone else had left, he was still there.

Suddenly, I felt embarrassed, that *we*, the emergency response team, as well-intentioned as we may have been, had been the intruders. We had burst in on this family, made a ruckus, broke the patient's ribs, declared him dead, and then disappeared as suddenly as we had arrived. We had never once attempted to try to understand anything more about this man other than the basic medical facts we needed to try to resuscitate him. Our involvement, unlike the surgeon's, felt unwelcome.

I quietly slunk out of the room and caught up to my team in the hall as they were making their way back to the emergency department. Their mood was jovial—after all, they hadn't spent as much time as I had analyzing what had just happened. They were talking about what food they wanted to order as a midnight snack. The man's cardiac arrest and subsequent death had just been one small part of another day for them. Patients die every day. Now it was back to the ER where plenty of new patients were waiting to be *greeted, treated, and streeted*, the depth of their relationships never deeper than a puddle after a light rain.

Early the next morning, I could barely stay awake as I drove home. What lingered in my mind was how the surgeon had managed to maintain a close bond with the patient and his family, even though he must have known at some point that the patient would not survive. How had he managed to do that? How had he not burned out? Was bonding with patients potentially the solution and not the problem? Would it be possible to form bonds like that as an emergency medicine doctor, *greeting, treating, and streeting* patients in rapid succession?

At that moment, any interest I'd had in emergency medicine disappeared. As clearly as I had known I had to go to medical school, I knew I would become a surgeon.

CHAPTER 6—What is Residency

After graduating medical school, newly minted doctors are expected to complete both an internship and a residency, in order to become board certified and practice medicine in the United States (or Canada). Internship refers specifically to the first year of residency.

But what exactly is *residency*? Good question. Technically, after graduating medical school, one is a doctor. Despite four intense years of med school, new grads don't yet know how to actually *be* doctors. They've spent two years studying in lecture halls and two years watching other people be doctors, but new grads haven't actually practiced any medicine ... yet. That's what residency is for. It provides a supervised environment for new doctors to learn how to practice medicine.

Residents are called *residents* because it is expected that they are at the hospital so much that they basically live there, figuratively (and sometimes literally) becoming *residents* of the hospital. While working at the hospital, they participate in every aspect of patient care, tailored to the specialty they are training in. In surgery, this includes things like doing rounds on post-operative patients, seeing new consults, preparing patients for surgery, discharging patients, changing dressings, taking out stitches, chest tubes, and other surgically placed drains from patients, writing an endless number of daily progress notes, reading thick surgical textbooks, preparing presentations, and of course, learning to operate. It's definitely not *Grey's Anatomy*.

In reality, the to-do list, referred to as *scut work* because it is tedious, time consuming, and without glory, is endless. There is always more that needs to be done. No one will ever clap you on the shoulder and congratulate you on how well written your progress note was. Just as a soldier is expected to make their bed after waking, residents are simply expected to get the scut work done.

The alcohol in the wound is that, during this time, residents are paid a nominal salary—just enough to cover living expenses, as well as the minimum loan repayment amount required to stay out of jail. Oh yeah, I forgot to mention—the minute you graduate med school, the government wants to be repaid those hundreds of thousands of dollars you borrowed to *go to* med school. *Stat.* They really don't care that you're technically still in training for another three to seven years. They want their money.

As painful as these years are, the scut work and years of residency training are critical. They are the final opportunity for the system to create safe and effective physicians by teaching young doctors how, at the very least, not to damage other human beings, before they are unleashed and begin practicing on the general public. This education comes at a price, though, and that price is freedom.

Residency programs vary in length, depending on specialty. The shortest is three years (internal medicine and family medicine) and the longest is seven years (neurosurgery). General surgery residency lasts for five years. Five ... very ... long ... years. Aside from duration, the intensity also varies between specialties. Psychiatry residencies, for example, are much less intense than those for general surgery and neurosurgery. All other specialties fall somewhere in between. As tough as residency is, the first challenge is getting accepted into a residency program. You'd think that getting into med school is the hardest part. It's not. Every step of the medical journey becomes tougher and more competitive. Fortunately, surgeons have a reputation for thriving on competition, and I was no exception.

I was accepted into my top-choice program, a Level 1 trauma center in Phoenix, Arizona. Having grown up in California, I was initially concerned about the scorching hot summers, but I quickly realized this would not be a problem, since I would be spending all of my time within the confines of the hospital, which—like every building in Phoenix—is air-conditioned year-round.

That spring, I graduated from med school in Kansas City. Everyone's parents were in attendance and just like in college, everyone wore caps and gowns and lined up on bleachers while various notable people gave long-winded speeches. And then, just when it seemed like it would never end, each graduate was called up, one by one, and we were given our diplomas.

My parents, especially my mom—who could not stop beaming—were overcome with joy at my accomplishment. It felt great to make my parents happy.

CHAPTER 7—Intern Year

I was an intern now. It was four-thirty a.m., and the sky was pitch black and the air cool outside. I was grateful, because later, the temperature would be over 110 degrees. I even shivered a little bit as I walked from my apartment to my car. I took a shortcut across a patch of grass, and some of the freshly cut pieces stuck to my shoes. I looked up at the clear dark sky and noticed a sliver of moon getting ready to retire for the day. No birds were flying overhead, there were no birds to fly; even they weren't up yet.

Still sleepy, I got into my car. My body ached with fatigue. Normally I am a morning person, but this was too early, even for me. It felt like I went to bed only a few hours ago. I put my key into the ignition and briefly considered walking back to my apartment, getting back into my warm bed, and going back to sleep. This thought was curtailed by the familiar *ding ding ding* telling me that my car door was still open, urging me to make a decision: get going or get out. I closed the door, turned the key, and my car roared to life. I envied its vigor this early in the morning.

As I pulled out of my parking spot, the guttural roar of the engine sliced through the quiet stillness of the morning. Each morning, I imagined the sound of my car's engine was the first noise that would begin the rest of everyone else's day, a signal to the still-sleeping city. I was a modern-day rooster.

I eased my car out onto the main road. From there it was a straight shot down a two-lane road to the freeway, which would take me almost the rest of the way to the hospital.

By the time I got on the freeway I was a little bit more awake, and I pretended my car was a rocket ship and the freeway onramp was my launch pad. I rapidly accelerated, feeling more invigorated now. I felt my car grip the ground as if it were an extension of my body. It carried me around each sweeping turn the empty freeway threw at me, back and forth. It was melodic and comforting, and if I hadn't been going so fast, I would have fallen back asleep.

As I turned off the freeway toward the hospital, anxiety began to set in. My eighteen minutes of tranquility were almost over. Once I got to the hospital, the rest of my day would be an all-out assault on my senses. The hospital is like a circus; it's bright, it's loud, it smells, and everyone is dressed in costumes playing their role. This was the last part of my day that belonged just to me. As soon as I left the solitude of my car, I would be at the beck and call of patients, attending surgeons, administrators, nurses, social workers, respiratory therapists, or whoever else.

I passed through the final intersection before I pulled up to the hospital. It was a five-way intersection, and worst of all, on one of its five corners, there was a bar, The Do Drop In, that never closed. This combination of confusing intersection and round-the-clock distribution of alcohol provided our trauma hospital with an endless stream of customers. Every morning as I drove through it, I checked all five directions to make sure I was not about to be slammed by a drunk driver. I wondered which came first: the hospital or the intersection? I wasn't sure if our *trauma* hospital was built here because of the proximity to such a confusing and dangerous intersection, or if the intersection was built after the hospital, as a way to drum up business. Frequent motor vehicle crashes were one of our daily (and nightly) specials. The level of a driver-turned-patient's intoxication increased exponentially as the night wore on.

The hospital parking garage was almost entirely empty so early in the morning. It took me eighteen minutes to get here. The fastest I've ever made it has been eleven minutes. I used to race for a personal best, until I got pulled over. I was going twice the speed limit on one of the surface streets. The officer that chased me down must have thought he'd caught an absolute maniac with the speed I was going. When he came up to my window, he saw me sitting there in my scrubs just shy of a mile from the hospital.

"Do you work at the hospital?"

"Yes," I said, feeling crestfallen as I calculated in my head how much I expected the ticket—and subsequent increase in my auto insurance—would cost me. *Just add it to my $250,000 dollar student loan tab*, I thought.

"Take care of our gunshot wounds and just slow down a little please," he said, and disappeared as quickly as he had appeared. I sat there, stunned. I didn't believe he'd let me go until after he had driven away. That morning, it took me twenty-one minutes to get to work.

I parked in my usual spot in the parking garage and turned my car off. I always hesitated before getting out. Every day, I considered for the second time, going back home, getting back into my warm bed, and going back to sleep.

No longer tired after my drive, I grabbed my bag off of the passenger seat and headed through the darkness. I entered through a discreet side door, away from the main entrance. Once inside I was only a few strides away from the resident work room.

The resident work room was a rectangular fluorescent room. The floor was made of an easy-to-clean plastic that resembles wood. The walls were white. On one of them hung a flat screen TV, which, without a cable connection, had no channels. Opposite the TV was a plastic green couch, a refrigerator, and a tiny coffee table. The far wall contained the main attraction: a long row of computers wirelessly connected to a large printer. Here was where we accessed patients' electronic medical records (EMR) and printed "The List"—patients we're responsible for during our twenty-four-hour shift. The entire room felt sterile, although it was anything but. We all knew where our feet had been: wading through pooled blood in the trauma bay, standing at the bedside of a patient with explosive diarrhea, or beneath the mouth of a patient who has just thrown up on us. Then, what did we do? Tracked it all back to the resident work room where we ate lunch, wrote notes, and tried to rest.

There were four rooms with beds—not to be confused with "bedrooms" like the one I'd just left—attached to the resident work room. Still, I found the overnight resident, Kyle, and a med student asleep. Although he was only a year ahead of me in residency, Kyle was several years older than me, owing to a stint in the Navy. Whenever I asked him what being in the Navy was like, he told me that N-A-V-Y stood for "Never Again Volunteer Yourself," and then changed the subject.

Kyle was sitting at the bank of computers with his head down on his folded arms, and the med student was lying on the couch with his eyes closed, breathing heavily. I couldn't blame them. They'd been in the hospital for twenty-four hours straight, and they wouldn't be able to go home until we had finished morning rounds. Tomorrow morning, it would be me asleep at the computers.

I walked over to Kyle and grabbed his right shoulder, gently shaking him awake, careful not to alarm him. Kyle was a year ahead of me in residency, which made him my senior resident. He abruptly popped his head up and looked around, briefly disoriented, while he figured out where he was.

"Morning," I said, as I tossed my bag down next to the couch, startling the med student, awake.

"Morning," he groggily replied, rubbing his eyes.

I pulled a chair up to the computer next to Kyle and logged in. "Anything new overnight?"

Coming to life, "Yeah, there are a few new patients I need to tell you about."

"Print me a list, will ya," I said, as I waited for the computer to verify my username and password.

The List contains the names and locations within the hospital of all of the patients that we are responsible for taking care of. Patients become a part of The List whenever they are admitted to the hospital or when another physician consults the surgery service. It's only once the patient is discharged (or dies), that they come off The List.

The List is a critical document. It rules our lives. Every morning, we print out The List, then spend the next hour looking up each patient's chart in the computer. Next to each patient's name, we write down important vital signs, lab values, and X-ray results in tiny letters and numbers.

The chief resident would be here in just over an hour and would want patient updates. There were thirty patients scattered throughout the hospital. If I was focused and quick, Kyle and I could see them all before the chief resident arrived. This allowed me roughly three minutes per patient, including travel time between rooms. In order to maintain my three-minute allotment per patient, I had to walk fast. I took the stairs so that I didn't get stuck waiting for an elevator.

When I walked into each patient's room, I knew exactly what information I needed from them. I gently woke each one up, then asked them the three general surgery questions: 1) How is your pain, 2) Have you eaten, and most important of all, 3) Have you pooped? (Between you and me, there is no better laxative than walking around the hospital first thing in the morning and asking people about their bowel movements. Nothing on this planet will make you more regular than that.)

Luckily, patients don't feel like chit-chatting this early in the morning, so I was able to escape each room in less than ninety seconds. *Yes!* But sometimes patients would give me circuitous answers or decide that now is the best time to ask for a comprehensive update of their entire hospital stay. I would explain that we'd come back later in the morning as a team and that we could chat more then. I've seen some other residents literally turn and walk out of the room while a patient is still talking, in order to stick to their tight morning schedule. I've always considered this to be rude and have never been able to do it myself.

At 6:46 a.m., I was exactly one minute late to meet up with Kyle and the chief resident, Brandon, in the Intensive Care Unit (ICU). Brandon was ready for us to give him updates. Kyle and I ran through The List, with the addition of the morning's lab results and our brief physical exams. Brandon would then use the information to formulate a plan of care for each patient.

Later that morning, he would present each plan to the attending surgeon. If Kyle and I had given him accurate information, we made him look good. If, in our haste, Kyle and I overlooked important details, then Brandon would look naive and uninformed. In turn, Kyle and I would look bad. Residents are kind of like garbage collectors—if we did our job well, nobody would know or care; if we messed it up, it would be very obvious to everyone and we would be in trouble. It was an un-winnable game, at least until later on in residency.

I pulled up a chair next to Brandon and Kyle. Brandon looked at me and then at his watch. *Oh, come on, man, I was* one minute *late.* In a hospital, though, everything has to be precise. Especially for a surgeon.

Over the next thirty minutes, we discussed each patient on The List. Kyle and I both squinted to read our tiny handwritten notes. Every so often, Brandon asked follow-up questions. When I didn't know the answer, it felt like a hot poker was being jabbed into my ribs. Shame, yes, but also a supremely unpleasant feeling not to know something I should.

"The patient in room 515, what day were antibiotics started?" Brandon asked me.

Uhhh … I glanced at Kyle, who silently shook his head. "I'm not sure," I said, as the familiar burning sensation arose.

Brandon shook his head. "Find out! You need to know these things."

Shortly thereafter, Brandon stopped me again. "How much came out of Mr. Smith's nasogastric tube after it was placed in the ER?"

Mr. Smith was one of the patients Kyle admitted overnight. He didn't tell me how much had come out, and I had forgotten to ask. Again, I glanced at Kyle, who kept his head down and pretended to examine his List.

The burning poker dug a little deeper between my ribs. I replied (again), "I'm not sure." The only worse response on my part would have been to make up a number. Residents would be fired for doing that.

Brandon set his List down on the desk and turned to face me. I braced myself.

"These are people's lives that we are giving you the privilege of taking care of. This is sloppy work." He glared at me. "Do you want to be a sloppy doctor?" His face registered a look somewhere between disapproval and disgust. "Why bother teaching you to operate if you can't even take care of post-op patients properly?" There was a long silence while he made a note on his clipboard. I held my breath until he sighed. "By the time you graduate, I want you to be someone that I would let take care of my family. Right now, you couldn't be further from that."

I felt disheartened, as though all my hard work had been discounted. Whenever I had the correct answers, I never heard "good job" or "atta boy." I was in a position now where not knowing could be deadly. Literally.

My face flushed, and I hoped it didn't show. All I could think was *"Fuck you!"* It hurt to be talked down to like this, especially when I'd worked so hard and jumped through so many hoops to get where I am. Med students stood behind me and witnessed this exchange. I was supposed to be their leader, but how could I muster up the charisma, much less confidence, to lead after this verbal lashing? At this moment, the chief resident felt like my worst enemy.

By the time we finished running The List, the guilt trip was over. Brandon looked at me and said—in lieu of an apology— "That's why it's a five-year program." He checked his watch and added, "Just enough time for a quick breakfast." I felt like a yo-yo, but we were friends again. Sort of.

On our first day of residency, during orientation, one of the attending surgeons, our new boss, had come in to talk to us. He was a tall, fit, older man dressed smartly in an immaculate suit. He exuded confidence. Being impressionable as we were at the time, he was someone we wanted to be like as soon as we saw him. I didn't know who he was, but I knew he was important by the way everyone immediately grew quiet and gave him their undivided attention. I was excited to hear what he had to say.

"I am Dr. Diaz. You are here to learn to become surgeons and *we* [the attendings] are here to teach you how. We aren't here to be friends. We don't want to be your friends. We already have enough friends. You're here to work and learn, and that is it."

With that, he left as abruptly as he had appeared.

After our quick breakfast, we headed to the preoperative holding area to meet up with the attending surgeon, Dr. Rostami, and the first patient we would operate on that day. It had only been a few hours since I woke up, and I'd already gotten so much done. I thought about how people who weren't residents were just now taking their first couple sips of coffee and preparing to begin their day. They still hadn't even gone to work yet. And once they did, they'd be home again before me. I allowed myself to feel some envy.

After we checked in with the attending surgeon and introduced ourselves to the patient, we headed over to *the board* which lists all of the scheduled surgical cases for the day. Here, our chief divided them up, assigning the big complex cases to higher level residents and smaller, less complex ones to lower levels. As an intern, it would be my duty to ensure that I had made headway on my scut work before returning to the O.R. to operate. Today, my scut work was not that bad, and I expected I'd be back by mid-morning. If I had been anything but a surgical resident, I would have taken my time getting through the scut work and never returned to the O.R. That would force the chief or another upper-level resident to do the small cases in my absence. This would piss them off, because by that stage, they'd mostly grown bored of the little cases and preferred to spend their time on the big ones. That's what separated surgical residents from other residents. Even if the reward for completing your work was more work, we'd still get it done in a timely fashion. That is the surgical way.

CHAPTER 8—Harder Than I Thought

When I first started intern year, I thought I was hot stuff. I was a newly minted doctor and figured I already knew most of what I needed to know. Cementing that notion, I finally got to wear a full-length white coat that came down nearly to my knees (medical students wear short white coats that end at their waist). In my mind, residency existed just to help me fine tune all the knowledge I'd acquired during the previous four years of medical school. I had made it through med school, done well on my clinical rotations, and achieved coveted scores on exams. I knew it all. Or so I thought.

One morning, while everyone was operating and I was working on my scut work, I went to check on a patient who was located in the medical intensive care unit (ICU). In the room with me was the patient's twin sister, sitting in a chair at the patient's bedside, holding her sister's hand. Both were about sixty years old. I can't remember exactly why the patient was in the hospital, but at this point, she was only semi-conscious and not really aware of either one of us.

As I was evaluating the patient, her twin sister began asking me questions and talking to me. Nothing out of the ordinary. Then all of a sudden, she stopped talking. I finished what I was doing and looked up at the twin sister and noticed that her face had become distorted. I asked if she was okay, to which she gave the gurgled reply, "Something is wrong, something is wrong, I think I am going to have a seizure!"

"Seizure …" I thought to myself, "I know how to treat a seizure—give Lorazepam." I considered the impending seizure as if it was a looming test question. I wondered, "But how much Lorazepam? And how to administer it?" I didn't know. Med school exam questions didn't usually ask about practical things like the doses of different drugs.

I looked up. The patient's twin sister had fallen to the ground and was now having a full on, arms and legs jerking, tonic-clonic seizure.

"Oh, shit."

I racked my brain, trying to figure out how much of the drug I needed to give and how to give it, "She probably won't be able to swallow a pill," I thought. But there was another problem that I wasn't even aware of yet. The twin sister wasn't a patient herself. I had no way of prescribing her medications, even if I did decide on the dose. We used an electronic medical record which is a computer-based system that contains every patient's medical records. Through this system we can click on patient's names and electronically order medications for them. But since she wasn't a patient, her name wouldn't be listed in the computer system anywhere for me to click on ...

I stood there watching her seize, growing more and more frantic. "Why wasn't a nurse or someone showing up and helping me?"

I poked my head out of the room and realized we were in a remote part of the ICU, and no one was really near us. I turned and looked back at the lady on the floor and noticed that her face had started to turn a shade of blue.

"Not good. Really not good." I felt time running out, I had to do something fast. But what?

I was hesitant to leave her there on the floor seizing and turning blue, but I needed help. I glanced at the patient and then down the hallway several times. There was still no one else around. Finally, I made up my mind that the best shot for this patient would be if I ran to get help.

I bolted down the hallway and quickly encountered a nurse doing something. "Call code blue! The family member of the patient in that room is having a seizure and turning blue!"

The nurse, unfamiliar with who I was (the new hotshot doctor, how could she not know!), continued what she was doing without looking up, unwilling to participate in my obvious hysteria. "The family member is having a seizure?" she casually repeated back to me. "We don't call code blues for that."

Running out of ideas I stammered, "Yeah, but we need to do something, she's turning blue and could die!" My panicked coaxing did little to change the outcome of our brief conversation. Maybe she was new also?

Growing more frantic, I looked around, hoping to lay eyes on someone else who could help me. There was no one. Why was this place a ghost town right at that moment?

Frustrated and afraid, I quickly moved on. Suddenly it occurred to me, I knew where I could find help. I calculated that the surgical ICU (SICU) team was in the middle of their morning rounds in the ICU next door. They were my people, surgeons. They would help me!

I ran through the double doors separating the two units. When I emerged on the other side, to my dismay, I didn't see the SICU team. "Where are they?" I mumbled under my breath, as I grew more frantic.

I ran up to the first nurse I saw and rapidly and breathlessly, barely comprehensibly, asked where the SICU team was. She gave me a concerned sideways look, then pointed and said, "On the other side of the SICU finishing rounds, why?" Without answering her question, I broke out into a run in the direction she had pointed.

Less than five minutes earlier, I had considered myself a hotshot new doctor. Now I was running through the SICU, sweat dripping down my forehead, searching for someone to help me. The reality of how much I had yet to learn—and how minimally useful I was as a doctor—was setting in. My pride had gone completely out the window. If I had stopped to think about it, I probably would have felt like I had been punched in the stomach and had the wind knocked out of me, but at that moment all I wanted to do was get help for this person.

I finally found the SICU team huddled in a large group outside a patient's room. One of the residents was standing in front of the team, reading lab values off of a sheet of paper. I was hesitant to interrupt, but I had no choice. I inserted myself between the resident and his audience. All eyes were now on me.

Out of breath I said, "I need help! There is a patient in the MICU who is having a seizure and turning blue!"

"Where's the MICU team?" came the SICU attending physician, Dr. Periera's voice, from within the crowd of scrubs.

"I have no idea. I couldn't find anyone." Then I added, "It's actually not a patient, it's the family member of one of the patients."

"What?" came Dr. Periera's voice, confused.

"Come with me!" I urged, and briskly led the group of people back across the SICU, through the double doors into the MICU, to the patient's room. Considering how long it had taken me to find help, I expected to find the patient's twin sister on the floor, cold and dead. My mind was racing. I felt guilty, I was barely out of medical school and my incompetence had already caused a patient's family member to die. I started to panic more.

To my shock, that was not what we found. By the time we arrived back at the room, the patient's twin sister—the one I imagined dead—was sitting in a chair at the patient's bedside. She was sipping out of a cup with a straw, held by the patient's nurse, who was kneeling on the floor next to her. She looked a little bit pale with a couple beads of sweat on her forehead, the only signs that she had ever been in any distress. Otherwise, she looked well. Not seizing, not blue, and certainly not dead. Staring at the scene in front of me, I heard the SICU attending Dr. Periera behind me ask sarcastically, "Is this the seizing lady?"

Embarrassed, my face flushed, I turned around and faced the group whose rounds I had interrupted. I felt like an idiot. Through the corners of my eyes, I thought that I could see a few smirking faces in the crowd.

"Yes ..." I trailed off for a moment, still a little bit stunned. "She was seizing, I saw

her ..."

"Okay, well everything looks under control now, we are going to finish up our rounds," Dr. Periera said. And then to her team, "C'mon guys, let's get back to the SICU and get done!" And with a wave of her arm, she led the crowd back through double doors and to the SICU, leaving me standing there bewildered.

Confused, I remained fixed in place, staring at the patient's twin sister, who just moments before, I had seen writhing on the floor. Now she was comfortably sitting in a chair, drinking water. After a few seconds I sensed someone at my side. I turned to find one of the MICU physicians standing next to me.

"What happened?" I asked, offering no description of the events that had transpired. I had a feeling he already knew.

"Pseudoseizures, man. They both have a history of it," he said, grinning and gesturing to the patient and the twin sister. "I think she did it the other day, too, when she was here visiting." Then, still grinning, he turned and walked away, leaving me standing there feeling like a useless pile of scrubs wearing a white coat.

Pseudoseizures, more formally known as psychogenic nonepileptic seizures, are not real seizures. They are unintentional movements that look like seizures. Why patients do it is not clear, but they are thought to be psychiatric in nature and are not dangerous. I should have known better, the way the twin sister told me she was about to have a seizure and the way she got onto the floor before writhing about was not characteristic of a true seizure in which someone abruptly loses consciousness. It was something I had yet to learn, and only experience could teach me.

I learned a valuable lesson that day, one that I would re-learn many times over throughout residency and beyond: Any time you start to get cocky, medicine will humble you. As embarrassing as it was, it was an important lesson to learn. Although I didn't realize it at the time, I was lucky to have learned it the way I did, without actually killing someone. Not everyone is so fortunate. Even now, years later, smarter, more skilled, and with more experience, I remember this lesson. Any time things are going well, and I begin to feel a little bit cocky, a little too confident, I slow down. Around every corner might be a patient lurking, ready to fool me with a pseudoseizure, or some other medical phenomena that I have yet to become familiar with, waiting to knock me back down a notch or two.

CHAPTER 9—The Tourists

J ust like in medical school, general surgery residents rotate through different surgical specialties. One of these specialties is trauma surgery. While rotating on trauma, we evaluated and resuscitated incoming trauma patients. We operated on them when necessary, and we took care of them while they recovered. All patients who have experienced physical trauma, whether or not they need an operation, get added to the Trauma List once they are admitted. The Trauma List was like The List I told you about, except this one was much longer. As the intern rotating on trauma, it was my job to ensure that the fifty or sixty patients on the TL were improving, so that they could be discharged from the hospital … before the list grew even larger.

One morning, as I went to check on one patient, Jimmy, he yelled at me, as if it was my fault he was injured and in pain. "I need more pain medicine! I'm in a lot of pain!" He was sitting up in his bed eating breakfast, shouting at me between bites of syrup-drenched pancakes. His mother sat silently in a chair next to his bed, wiping Jimmy's mouth between bites, and another woman—his sister?—sat in a chair at the foot of the bed.

Jimmy was a bearded, overweight thirty-seven-year-old who had been involved in a head-on motor vehicle collision ("MVC," as we refer to them) on the highway. Miraculously, despite not wearing his seatbelt, the only injuries he had sustained were four rib fractures and lots of bruises. He didn't need surgery. Ninety-nine percent of the time, rib fractures heal on their own. In the meantime, it was the trauma team's job to take care of him

70

until he was well enough to be discharged.

"Your accident was six days ago," I told him. "You broke four ribs. Like we discussed before, I can't take all the pain away, but I can make it manageable," I replied, trying to be calm and firm without inciting an argument.

"But it hurts so BAD!" he barked back at me. He waved his fork to emphasize his point; this dragged strings of sticky syrup across the front of his hospital gown. "The medicine you are giving me isn't working, I want more of the one that begins with a 'D'! That's the only one that works!"

The one that begins with the letter 'D' is 'Dilaudid', a synthetic opioid that is ten times stronger than morphine. As the opioid crisis in America continued to surge, opioid medications were villainized in the media, and there was a lot of pressure on doctors to limit their use. The media failed to publicize this type of interaction, which physicians encounter daily, in which patients demand opioids for their pain. Finding the line between humanely relieving suffering and being irresponsible was left up to me.

"Look," I began, trying my best to sound empathetic even as my frustration grew, "you want to go home, don't you?"

"Yes," he shot back, eyeing me skeptically.

"Well, you won't have an IV at home and therefore we can't send you home if you are still using IV pain medications. That's why we are trying to wean you off of them," I replied, trying to reason with him.

What I had really wanted to tell him was how lucky he was compared to the others who had been in the same car wreck—all of whom had only recently been released from the ICU—but strict patient privacy protection laws prevented me from doing so.

Before he could say anything further, his mouth full of pancakes, his mother glared at me. "So, you're just going to let him suffer?" she said, contemptuously, as she wiped away more syrup and pancake crumbs from her adult son's chin.

I tried again, "I understand he's in pain. As I have tried to explain before, we cannot take *all* of the pain away, but I will do the best we can to make it tolerable." I felt a surge of adrenaline. We weren't getting anywhere, and there were other patients who were waiting to speak with me.

The mother crossed her arms and flashed a haughty look at me, but she didn't say anything more. I used her momentary silence to try to move the conversation forward. "What's really important is that he gets out of bed and works with the physical therapist. That will help prevent him from getting blood clots, pneumonia, and losing strength while he is reco—"

Uninterested in what I had to say about preventing blood clots and pneumonia, his sister cut me off, "What about his blood sugars? How have they been running?" From the moment he had arrived at the hospital, Jimmy had been surrounded by caring family members who doted over him nonstop. He was luckier than most.

"His blood sugars have been fine. This morning it was 101."

His sister gasped, and then feigning disbelief, "That's too high! He's pre-diabetic, don't you know that!? Why aren't you doing a better job of controlling his blood sugars?!"

Trying to avoid sounding dismissive, I calmly replied, "A blood sugar of 101 is O.K. while he is here in the hospital. He will need to visit with his primary care doctor once he is out of the hospital to adjust his medications to get them lower than that."

I felt like I was on trial. Meanwhile, Jimmy, who had just finished stuffing his face with pancakes, orange juice, and a bowl of cereal, sat in front of us surrounded by candy wrappers and the remains of other snack foods that his family had been bringing him non-stop. Every day I told them to stop, but every day they continued.

My pulse quickened. *If you were so concerned about his blood sugar ...* I thought to myself, fighting the urge to say it out loud. Instead, I smiled at the three of them and rounded out the encounter with, "Do you have any other questions?"

They all shook their heads distractedly. They were no longer interested in talking to me. Jimmy had finished eating and was now performing burps for his mother and sister, who laughed as though Jimmy were a Las Vegas comedian.

I forced a smile and said, "Well, if anything comes up, don't hesitate to let one of the nurses know. They always know how to get hold of me." With that, I left the room and went to the next patient's room.

One of the third-year medical students began his carefully rehearsed patient presentation, "Mrs. Tanaka is a thirty-two-year-old female who was recently downgraded from the intensive care unit after being involved in a head-on motor vehicle collision six days ago resulting in multiple spine fractures ..."

The medical student finished his summary. We entered the room, evaluated the patient, updated her on her progress, and then moved on to the next patient, repeating the process again.

"Mr. Tanaka is a thirty-four-year-old male who was recently downgraded from the intensive care unit after being involved in a head-on motor vehicle collision six days ago sustaining a complex pelvic fracture complicated by hemorrhagic shock that is now resolved ..."

Then we went in the room, evaluated the patient, updated him on his progress, and moved on to our last patient.

"Mrs. Yamamoto is a fifty-seven-year-old female who was recently downgraded from the intensive care unit after being involved in a head-on motor vehicle collision six days ago, sustaining a traumatic brain injury and tibial plateau fracture ..."

As we exited the room, my pager went off. It was Jimmy's nurse paging me. He wanted more pain medication, and his family had more questions. I took a deep breath and walked back down the hall toward his room. As I walked, I thought about how these four patients were all related.

Mr. and Mrs. Tanaka came from modest means and were recently married in their home country of Japan. They decided to take a honeymoon to America. They saved their money and planned the trip of a lifetime: They planned to see as many of the main attractions as they could, like the Golden Gate Bridge, Disneyland, Yosemite, Yellowstone, the Grand Canyon, and probably many more. Because they didn't speak English, they hired a Japanese tour guide, Mrs. Yamamoto, to help them get around.

Their two weeks in America eventually drew to a close, and on their final day, just before dawn on a Thursday morning, six days prior to this day, Mrs.

Yamamoto drove the Tanaka's to the airport. They would have plenty of time to get through security and board their flight back home to Japan. They were on the empty freeway, less than fifteen minutes from the airport, when a drunk driver speeding the wrong way on the freeway smashed head-on into them, crippling and nearly killing the three of them. The drunk driver of course, was Jimmy.

The same Jimmy who was summoning me back to his room to tell me how much pain he was in, while he ate pancakes and was doted on by his caring family—and they basically accused me of neglecting him.

The Tanakas, on the other hand, were alone, thousands of miles from home, and had much worse injuries. Despite this, they never once complained. After each update I gave them, they thanked me, and never once made me feel like they were questioning the quality of the care I was providing for them.

That morning, I had just finished telling the Tanakas that our case manager had been able to arrange a flight back to Japan for them. Although they would still require further care in a hospital, now that they were out of the intensive care unit, and *stable*, their traveler's insurance demanded that they be transferred back to Japan to finish their treatment. The hospital had arranged for them to fly commercial. I thought about how uncomfortable they would be on such a long flight sitting upright in the rigid airline seats wearing their neck and back braces. Meanwhile, Jimmy would be in our hospital, sleeping comfortably, looking forward to morphine shots, delicious meals, and spending the day hanging out with his family. It seemed unfair.

As much as the circumstances of what had happened bothered me, I didn't hate Jimmy, and I didn't allow the situation to influence the quality of medical care I provide for him. To keep things simple, I decided early on that I would always provide every one of my patients with high quality care, no matter what. I didn't *like* Jimmy, but that was irrelevant. He needed my help. Everyone makes mistakes.

Every patient has different emotional needs. Some have more emotional needs than others, which I discovered is usually the result of fear. Being in a hospital is scary. Patients aren't always able to communicate that they are scared, and instead, their fear can manifest itself in a variety of different ways. Maybe Jimmy and his family were just projecting their fear onto me by being skeptical of the care I was providing. It was, and is, my job as a physician to not only provide care for my patient's physical problems, but also empathy and compassion for their emotional ones as well.

As my experience in trauma surgery continued, I would have more experiences like this one. Sometimes I would have to care for both the police officer that was shot and the suspect that fired the shot. Or a woman whose husband beat her face to a pulp, as well as the husband who was nearly killed by her retaliatory knife wound. Dichotomies like this exist in trauma surgery all the time. The details that bring a trauma patient to the hospital can be intriguing, sad, and occasionally, even funny.

CHAPTER 10—Burn Baby Burn

My intern year ended without fanfare, and soon I was a second-year resident. Second year was similar to intern year in the sense that we were still considered *junior* residents. However, by now, I had begun to understand how to be efficient in the hospital. I could see patients, write orders, change dressings, and have my notes done in a tenth of the time that it had taken me just months earlier. Rotating through different surgical specialties would continue for the remainder of residency, and my next rotation was in the burn unit.

Most hospitals do not have burn units. Each region of the United States has a single hospital with a highly specialized burn unit; that hospital treats burn patients from throughout the region. The hospital where I was a resident did not have a burn unit. Therefore, I had to travel across town to a separate hospital that was the receiving burn unit for a large swath of the American Southwest.

Up to this point in residency, I'd only had one encounter with a burn patient, and it was on my first day of intern year, July first. A fifty-six-year-old woman had been having chest pain at work, so a co-worker volunteered to take her to the hospital. Halfway to the hospital, her chest pain worsened, and she became unresponsive. Her co-worker pulled over, got her out of the car, laid her flat on the pavement, and began doing chest compressions while he waited for help to arrive. By the time the ambulance got to them, her heart had restarted, but she had third degree burns on her back, neck, arms, and legs from lying on the summer-hot Phoenix pavement for a mere nine minutes.

My first day in the burn unit was a Monday. At first glance, the unit resembled any other: brightly lit large patient rooms with floor to ceiling sliding glass doors, which all wrapped around a central front desk area with computers. This ICU, however, was more chaotic than the ones I'd seen before. All hospitals feel a bit like a parallel universe; here, I felt like I'd entered another dimension entirely. Almost immediately, my senses were overwhelmed. Phones were constantly ringing and being answered, orders being shouted from one person to another, doors opening and closing, carts being wheeled every which way, the endless beeping of monitors, the sound of typing, printers printing (and then immediately jamming, followed by cursing), charts being smacked down onto tables, exasperated sighs of nurses, and the occasional shriek of a patient. There was a constant movement of people all around me, and the ever-present glow of artificial bright white fluorescent light buzzed and flickered every now and then.

I walked over to the desk and introduced myself to a large man who was sitting at the nurses' station. He was answering the phones, which rang nonstop. He'd ask the caller to hold, and then shout in the general direction of the unit things like, "Stacy! It's lab calling for you on line one with a critical result!"

Between setting one phone down and picking up another, he nodded at me and pointed at two people wearing scrubs sitting at near the end of the long desk to his left. It was the first of the month, when residents typically change rotations, and apparently, he was used to lost newbies like me.

I went to the end of the desk. Two stressed-looking women in green scrubs were squinting at computer screens and typing at a pace I didn't think was humanly possible. I stood on the other side of the desk and cleared my throat. One of them looked up, and I introduced myself, "Hey, I'm Ryan, the new resident for this month."

The first woman immediately stopped typing and her face morphed into a smile. "Thank God you're here, we need all the help we can get! There's so much to do!" she exclaimed.

"Great, how can I help?" I replied, happy to be welcomed.

"We just finished rounding and I need to get these orders in before cases start." Then, noticing that I was wearing dress clothes she added, "Do you have scrubs yet? You need scrubs. We need all the hands we can get in the O.R." Then, turning back to her computer, she added again, "There's just *so much* to do!"

I was still wearing a shirt and slacks, because I wanted to make a good impression on my first day. "No one has given me any scrubs yet. They just sent me over here after I got my badge."

The second woman now looked up at me. And down again. From the way she spoke, I could tell that she was the more senior of the two, the *burn chief.* "You need to get into some scrubs ASAP. I'm going to need you to put in a line in Room 3," she said, as she pointed. "Then when you finish, I need you to help in the O.R." As she said this, she stood up. "Oh, and by the way, I'm Erin, your chief resident for the next month."

Hearing this, the other woman added, "And I'm Sarah, one of the other junior residents rotating with y'all this month."

I changed into scrubs, then looked at my feet. Damn. I was still wearing dress shoes, because I hadn't expected to operate that day. I hate wearing dress shoes with scrubs. I think it looks goofy, because dress shoes are so formal, and scrubs look as informal as pajamas. I especially hate wearing dress shoes if I'm going to do something that might get them dirty. I hadn't brought a change of shoes because secretly I'd been hoping to have the afternoon off after orientation. I should have known better.

I walked back to the front desk clutching my folded dress clothes. When I got there, Erin looked down at my shoes and frowned, "You're going to want to wear shoe covers."

"Thanks," I replied, unenthusiastically.

"Let me show you where you can put your stuff," she added, leading me to an overcrowded break room.

"This is where everyone puts their stuff and eats food, if they brought any. If you didn't, there's a cafeteria in the basement, but I don't recommend it unless you are literally starving to death."

I tucked my stuff away in a corner where it was out of sight. As I did so, Sarah reminded me, "That patient in Room 3 still needs a line. The O.R. is still being turned over, so if you could get that line in ASAP that would be great."

"Great!" My spirits lifted as I re-calibrated from the anticipation of enjoying an afternoon off to the anticipation of working in the ICU. Also, I was eager to put in a line.

"I'll show you where everything you need is, and then you're on your own." Then, as an afterthought she added, "You've put in lines before, right?"

Trying to sound confidant, "Yes, of course." This was a partial lie.

"Good."

She led me to a typical hospital supply room with long shelves overflowing with identical appearing white packages. We grabbed everything I would need and then she pointed me in the direction of Room 3, adding, "Holler if you need help." Then, she disappeared.

As I walked to Room 3, I thought that no matter what, I would not take her up on her offer to help. Doing a procedure, especially as a resident, is a thing of pride. A way to show off your skills and appear capable. Especially now that I was a second-year resident, I was desperate to prove my worth. This was an opportunity to demonstrate my competence. I would not blow this.

Line, or *central line*, is a special IV that is larger and longer than the ones nurses put in your arm. It's long enough to travel down the patient's vein all the way to their heart, where blood flow is greatest. Central lines can be required for a number of reasons, for example, when the doctors can't insert a normal IV, when patients need to receive medications that are toxic to smaller veins, or when they need dialysis. In the case of Room 3, the patient needed a central line for all of these reasons.

With all the supplies I had just gathered cradled in my arms, I used my hip to nudge open to the door and stepped in. Lying motionless on the bed was an unconscious man, connected to a ventilator that was breathing for him. I could barely tell he was human. He was covered from head to toe in white bandages that concealed what I was sure were horrific burns. The few parts of his body that were visible were swollen like the Michelin Man or the Pillsbury Dough Boy. His skin was stretched so tight that it looked as if it might burst open at any moment.

The bandages and swelling were going to make it exceedingly difficult and more dangerous to insert the line. Aside from the beeping of the various life support machines, the room was quiet. I was suddenly aware that I was completely alone with this very ill patient. Furthermore, the truth was, I had never placed a central line completely on my own before, usually only under direct supervision.

There are three locations on the human body where access to the invisible deep central veins are possible: the groin, the neck, or underneath the collar bone. The groin is the easiest and lowest risk, while underneath the collar bone is the most challenging and highest risk. The neck location sits somewhere in between. I set my supplies down on the bedside table and stood at the patient's bedside, examining him from head to toe. My eyes darted from his neck to his clavicle to his groin.

Mentally I made note that both sides of the patient's groin were covered with bandages and inaccessible. Not ideal. Next, I looked at his neck and noticed central lines already coming out of each side. A wave of relief washed over me. I thought Erin had made a mistake, maybe she didn't know the patient already had lines!

While I stood pondering this, the patient's nurse poked her head into the room. Seeing the supplies I had just set down, she smiled and cheerily said, "Oh good! You're here to put in a new line, right?"

"Yes, but it looks like he already has a central line," I said, puzzled.

She chuckled and then said, "Yes, he certainly does. Two, in fact."

She pointed at the one in his left neck. "This one is for dialysis," then moved her finger to the one in his right neck. "This one is for all of the medications he is on."

"But—" I started, still confused, "most of those medications can go through a normal peripheral IV … why does he need so many central lines?"

She chuckled again. "You're new here, aren't you?"

I nodded silently.

"As part of burn patients' initial resuscitation, they are given a massive amount of IV fluids, that's why their entire body swells up. See?" she said, gesturing toward the patient. "And when they become that swollen, there is no way to insert a peripheral IV. The only way to get IV access to give them medications is with central lines." She paused and looked at me to make sure she wasn't boring me, then continued. "Because these patients are so sick and here for so long, every week, we have to take out the old ones and put in new ones to try to minimize the chance of the line becoming infected. That's why he needs a new line today, the one in his left neck is getting old, it's been there for ten days already." Then, as quickly as she had appeared, she disappeared again leaving me alone with the patient and my thoughts.

I started to grow nervous that I had bitten off more than I could chew by agreeing to put in a new line on my own. Since this was my first day, and this was my first task, I didn't want to have to ask Erin to help me. I was eager to make a good first impression, that I was competent and capable. But if something bad happened, how competent would I seem then?

My mind, like Mentos added to a bottle of soda, began to rapidly fill up with these unhelpful thoughts, to the point where I thought my head might explode. *What if I couldn't get the line in like I had been asked to do? Worse yet, what if this patient started to die while I was placing the line? Would someone know to come help me? Would I have to scream for help? If I couldn't do this, would I get laughed out of the burn unit?* My palms began to sweat. *Maybe I should have told Erin I had never done this on my own before and asked for help.*

I felt irritated that I had allowed these counterproductive thoughts to enter my brain. I mustered all my strength and shifted my focus to mentally reviewing the steps to placing a central line. It was like a game of tug-o-war was taking place in my brain.

I had been eager to prove myself, and this was my chance.

Although inserting a central line is considered a basic procedure, it isn't always easy. And my assessment so far of this bloated, dying patient, covered in bandages, with only the location beneath his collar bone available for central line insertion, all but guaranteed this one would not be easy.

I stared at both of the patient's clavicles, trying to decide which side to attempt. I noticed multiple needle marks below both clavicles. Someone had already been trying and failed. Not good. I considered my options: I could immediately admit defeat, humble myself, and ask for help. I could try, fail, and *then* ask for help. Or worst of all, I could try, cause a complication and kill the patient, and then I'd have to ask for both help and forgiveness.

Worst-case scenarios ran through my mind. A devil appeared floating over my left shoulder and repeated the nagging inner monologue I had heard so many times before, "You're an imposter, you're not good enough, and can't do it. You didn't even pass anatomy the first time, how on Earth are you going to find the subclavian vein in this guy! You shouldn't even be here in the first place. The only reason you are is because the residency program director made a mistake by accepting you. She was in a hurry when she filled out the rank list, and she clicked your name by accident. She's probably waiting for a reason to fire you, and if you hurt this patient, she'll finally have one!" I started to sweat.

Then, an angel appeared on my right shoulder, "You've seen this done many times before. You've done it before. You can do this." And before I gave the devil a chance to counter, I began setting up all of my materials.

At least the patient is asleep and won't squirm, I told myself. After I had everything set up, I donned my sterile surgical gown and gloves, took a deep breath, and placed the sterile surgical drape over the patient.

Just as I was about to make my first attempt to insert the needle underneath the patient's collar bone, Erin poked her head in. "Everything okay in here?"

But before I could answer she went on, "They're done turning over the O.R. and wheeling in our next patient now. After you're done here, come join us. I'll see you in there shortly." She disappeared as suddenly as she had appeared.

I turned back to what I was doing and picked up my syringe, to which was affixed a long shiny needle. The needle was about four inches long. With my gloved hand I held it up, noticing the light glint off of it. To a bystander I must have looked like a mad doctor from an old science fiction movie about to turn a patient into a science experiment. The only thing missing was evil laughter.

I reached down and tried to feel anatomic landmarks that would help me blindly guide the long needle into the vein. Although collarbones are normally prominent, on this man, his were nearly impossible to find, because of how swollen he was. After digging my fingertips into his bloated shoulder several times, I found it. I took a deep breath, and then pushed the giant needle into his skin. Now underneath his skin, I directed the needle toward his clavicle. I pictured the vein just below the clavicle. Easy-peasy. I had to go just far enough under the clavicle to get into the vein, but not too far or I would puncture the lung. The patient was already in critical condition, and I didn't think that he had enough reserve left to survive a collapsed lung.

I held my breath and advanced the long needle. It came to a sudden stop as it scraped against the collar bone, like nails on a chalk board.

That's okay, I told myself, *you're just a little bit too high. No harm done. Just walk the needle down underneath the bone and you'll be in the vein.*

I retracted the needle slightly and made micro adjustments to its trajectory before I tried again. This time, the needle kept advancing forward, farther than before. I was now able to slide the needle underneath the bone, inching it closer to the vein ... but also closer to the lung just underneath.

I moved the needle a little bit farther than before and held my breath. I would know I'd contacted the vein when my syringe filled with blood. I glanced at the syringe. It was still empty. I pushed the needle a little bit deeper, feeling my sphincter tighten as more of the needle disappeared into the patient. Still nothing.

Each little bit that I advanced the needle without finding the vein risked the needle going too far and hitting the lung instead. That would collapse the lung and likely kill the patient.

I kept advancing the needle. Suddenly I realized that I had advanced the entire four inches of the needle into the patient. There was no more needle left to go and I had still not found the vein. I began to panic as I imagined the tip of the needle sitting inside of his lung. Sweat began bubbling up on my forehead and running down the side of my face, causing it to itch. I couldn't stop and scratch it now. With the entire needle buried in this guy's chest, and potentially his lung, I needed to focus.

I pulled the needle out and frantically looked up at the patient's monitor and checked his vital signs to see if he had any signs of a collapsed lung. To my relief, his oxygen level was unchanged. My sphincter unclenched. I had just dodged a bullet.

I had been able to insert the entire needle into the patient without hurting him. That restored my confidence and my resolve to get the line in. I pressed the needle into his skin and tried again. And again. And then again. No luck. I tried a few more times with similar results, each time growing less and less optimistic that I could do it.

I decided to put my tail between my legs and ask for help. I stuck my head out of the patient's room and scanned the scene outside. From where I was standing, I could see the desk where the residents worked. Erin was not there; she had gone the O.R. Instead, I saw Sarah, the other junior resident, still sitting at the computer typing.

"Sarah!" I whispered loudly in her direction, trying not to draw unwanted attention to me.

She looked up, and saw me covertly gesturing at her for help, and walked over.

"What's up?" she asked.

"I'm having trouble with this central line. Can you help me?"

"Okay," she said. "Let's see what's going on."

She stepped into the room with me, and we walked over to my setup. She noticed immediately that I had been repeatedly poking the patient's chest, trying to find the subclavian vein underneath the clavicle.

"Oh, shit!" she exclaimed. "Subclavian! I'm terrible at those. And this guy is ridiculously swollen too. I always just do neck or groin, why don't you just do that?"

I explained why not.

"Well, if you can't do it, I probably can't either. Just wait until Erin is done operating and ask her to do it."

I didn't want to do that. I wanted to get the line in before I went to the O.R., so that when Erin asked me how things had gone, I could nonchalantly say, "Fine." I wanted her first impression of me to be as a competent team member. But with how things were going and Sarah being unable to help, I didn't see any other way. Crestfallen and humbled, I took down the surgical drapes that I had set up and discarded the supplies that I had opened, all of which had remained unused except for the needle. Opened and no longer sterile, these supplies were useless other than to serve as further evidence of my failure.

As I stepped out of the patient's room, I heard a voice in my direction. It was the patient's nurse, "You get that line in?"

Avoiding eye contact, "No," I replied quietly. My cheeks flushed with shame.

I found my way to the operating room. I paused outside and remembered how Erin had advised me to wear shoe covers. I leaned against the wall and pulled the blue covers on over my dress shoes. My feet were starting to hurt from standing for so long. I had a feeling they'd be hurting a lot more by the end of the day.

I pushed open the door to the O.R., and a wave of heat hit me in the face. It was like taking a pizza out of the oven. Inside, a burn patient equally as swollen and unidentifiable as the one in 3 was lying on the operating room table, asleep. A crowd of people, including Erin, surrounded the patient. Everyone wore surgical gowns. I didn't want to draw attention to the news I was about to deliver, so I walked up and stood quietly next to her.

"Hey!" she said cheerily, shattering any hope I had at confidentiality, "You get that line in?"

I shook my head.

"How come?"

I explained what had happened and my numerous failed attempts.

"It's okay," she said, "central lines on these guys are tough. I'll give it a try when we're done here. By the end of the month, you'll be a pro."

Why was she being so nice? Was she faking it? In the back of her mind was she silently judging me, labeling me as useless? This is the type of paranoia surgical residency breeds.

"How can I help?" I asked, gesturing toward the patient on the table, eager to redeem myself.

"This patient had sixty-percent of his total body surface area burned off after a car accident. He was trapped inside when the car caught fire. We need to debride more of the dead skin to try to get it ready for skin grafting. Today we are going to work on the left side of his torso, and we could really use your help."

"It's really hot in here," I remarked. I suspected it wasn't just me who thought so. I glanced around the room and noticed that everyone was sweating profusely behind their masks, their surgical gowns concealing what I could only imagine was sweat drenched scrubs underneath.

She chuckled. "Tell me about it. It's not something you probably ever think about, but skin is essential for helping us stay warm. Since most of these patients' skin is missing, they can't maintain their body heat, so we have to do it for them, thus this room is heated to the high nineties. It really sucks for us, especially once we get our gowns on and start operating." She continued, "Especially since the electrocautery we use to cut away the dead tissue is also really hot." Then she added, thoughtfully, "It's ironic how we treat burns with more burns."

I nodded along, listening carefully.

She gestured to a door at the side of the operating room and added, "If you get light-headed, go in there and drink something. We keep that room cool, like a reverse sauna. Inside, there is a small refrigerator with drinks. We don't want you to pass out, and believe me, it happens all the time."

I certainly didn't want that to happen either, and I made a mental note to myself about the room. Still embarrassed that I had not been able to get the central line in like Erin had asked me to, I already worried that she thought I was a weak team member. I definitely wasn't going to add "unable to stay conscious during surgery" to my growing list of disappointments so far.

I scrubbed my hands and then took my place next to Erin on the patient's left side. She handed me the *Bovie*, a plastic instrument shaped like a pen with a button on the side that instantly heats the metal tip to a temperature high enough to cut through flesh like a lightsaber. She pointed to an area of charred flesh.

"Cut all of this away. While you work on there, I'll work up here. We're going to have to go fast. If we stay too long, the patient will get sick. He's going to bleed a lot while we do this, and despite the warm room temperature, he'll cool off. We have to be out of here in no more than two hours, so move fast!" She clicked the button on her Bovie and began to cut. I did the same, determined to make up for my previous failure by showing her I was useful in the O.R.

I cut and cut and cut. More than I ever had before in my life. Just when I thought there was no more dead tissue left to cut, there was more. With each stroke, the Bovie incinerated the patient's flesh, creating billows of hot smoke that wafted up into my face, easily permeating through my flimsy surgical mask. The smell of charred flesh entered my mouth, filled my lungs, and left my mouth filled with the smokey aftertaste of charred meat. I was sweating profusely, and I was parched.

I kept cutting, removing hunks of charred flesh, handing each piece to the scrub tech. At the end of the surgery, she would dispose of the dead tissue. I wondered if it ever ended up in the cafeteria. Maybe that's why Erin had told me not to eat there.

With each section of flesh we removed, the patient oozed blood from the healthy tissues underneath. Cumulatively, this resulted in significant blood loss, like Erin had warned me about. The blood pooled together and formed thick streams that blended together into rivers as it ran down the sides of the surgical drapes like a bloody waterfall. The blood splashed onto the floor and all over my shoe covers. I was glad I had worn them.

While I was trying to stop a patch of oozing with my Bovie, Erin turned to check on me. "Don't waste time doing that. Just put one of these on it and keep going," she said motioning to a piece of damp white gauze the scrub tech was holding in an outstretched hand. "It's a bandage soaked with chemicals that make the body's small blood vessels stop bleeding. Just lay it over the area that's oozing and keep working."

I nodded and took the dripping material from her. I laid it over the raw surface and returned to cutting. It looked like we were butchering the patient, hacking him to pieces. But Erin seemed to know what she was doing, so I followed her lead. While we cut, I thought about the classic surgical saying, "A chance to cut is a chance to cure." I wondered if that saying implied a one-to-one ration, because we were definitely doing a lot of cutting, and I hoped we were doing as much curing.

When we had finally finished removing all of the dead tissue and replacing it with the special bandages, I was soggy with sweat all the way down to my underwear. I glanced at the clock and noticed that only about an hour had elapsed. I was stunned by how slowly time had passed.

"Okay," Erin said, getting my attention, "Now we need to clean up and get out of here." She showed me how to remove the dressings we had placed to help slow the bleeding. By the time we had removed them all, I was suddenly aware that I was staring at a patient who was nearly completely skinless. I had never seen anything so horrible before in my life.

As if she had been reading my mind, Erin said, "Now we need to get it covered. We're going to use cadaver skin."

Uh ... Cadaver skin?!

On the back table, the scrub tech had been opening packages of thin flesh that had been defrosting in a basin of warm water. Erin fished a piece of the flesh out of the water and held it so that I could see. It was bunched up like a wet tissue. She placed the piece of skin down and carefully unrolled it, making sure not to tear it. After she had finished, it had become a rectangle about the size of an iPhone. Next, she showed me how to place it over an area of exposed flesh and use a stapler to secure it in place.

"Just like that," she said. "Try not to waste any, it's very expensive. I think each piece costs a few thousand dollars. In a week or so we will come back, take it all off and replace it."

"Why do we need to do that?" I naively asked.

"Because it's not *his* native skin and his body knows it. The cadaver skin will help keep the raw areas covered while they heal, but it will eventually fall off. Eventually, when he is ready, we will replace each piece with a skin graft from what he has left of his own skin."

I got busy doing exactly what she had just showed me: I fished clumps of rolled up cadaver skin out of the basin of water, unrolled them, and then tried to align them over raw surfaces on the patient. It was tedious work. Toward the end of the procedure, after we had gotten most of the wounds covered, it became like a sick arts and craft project, cutting pieces of skin so that they would perfectly cover the patches of still exposed raw surface.

Eventually, the anesthesiologist told us it was time to wrap things up. By the time we finished, we had gone only a little bit over our two-hour time limit. In total, we'd used forty-two pieces of cadaver skin to re-cover the patient's wounds. Multiply that times $2,000 for each piece, and we'd spent $84,000 for the cadaver skin alone.

Erin and I helped bundle the patient up in extensive white gauze dressings, which made him indistinguishable from the other patients in the burn unit. The second we finished, I tore off my surgical gown. My scrubs underneath were soaking sweat. I looked like I had just been pushed into a pool. I carefully peeled off my blood-soaked shoe covers and looked down at my shoes, disappointed to find that the cheap covers had not been able to hold back the relentless onslaught of blood that had come from the patient. My shoes were blood soaked and ruined.

Erin laughed and pointed out the obvious "You're going to need to get new shoes, I thought I told you to put on shoe covers!"

"You did … I did …" I stammered, too overheated and exhausted to elaborate.

I followed her into the cool-off room. She pulled two water bottles out of the fridge and handed me one. At that moment, the cold room felt like paradise.

"As soon as they turn this room over, we have another case," Erin said, cutting through my bliss and bringing me back to reality, "In the meantime, let's go see about that central line …" she said, leading me out of the O.R. and back to Room 3.

Standing back in Room 3, I watched silently as Erin inserted the central line. Neither of us ever mentioned it again.

On my second day in the burn unit, one of the patients I helped take care of was a woman in her thirties who had been trapped in a house fire with her daughter. Although her child had been severely burned, we expected that she would survive. The mother, on the other hand, had suffered much more extensive burns, and her outcome was less clear. The burns had consumed 80% of her body, including her entire face. As a result, her face had become charred and unrecognizable. We took her to the operating room and did the same as we did for yesterday's patient—only this time, we focused on her face. All the skin on her face had died, so we peeled off her entire face (yes, it was as gross as it sounds). I wondered to myself, if she survived, what kind of life would she have afterward?

Occasionally, the cause of the burns could be as horrific as the damage they caused. Aside from the usual house fires and people trapped in a burning vehicle, we took care of people who unknowingly lived next door to a meth lab. Another woman had been standing next to a propane tank when it exploded, and there were several young children who had reached up toward hot stoves and accidentally tipped a pot of boiling water onto themselves. Among all of this, there was "The Vape Incident."

"The Vape Incident" occurred when a young woman in her twenties had been using her vape while driving a large pick-up truck. One day, the vape exploded and spewed flaming hot liquids, which caused her pants to catch fire. In response, she tried to stop, drop, and roll. Except that the truck was still moving. She threw the door of her truck open, hurled herself out onto the pavement and rolled on the ground. The still-moving truck ran her over and broke her pelvis before it finally crashed into a tree.

When she arrived, she had third degree burns around her inner thighs and labia and a broken pelvis. Her back, legs, and arms were covered in serious road rash.

Besides horrific burns, the burn ICU also took care of patients with terrible wounds from other disease such as *necrotizing soft tissue infections* (flesh-eating bacteria) and *Steven Johnson Syndrome* (a life-threatening type of severe allergic reaction in which the patient's skin begins to slough off uncontrollably). Basically, our burn ICU took care of anything horrific that could happen to a person's skin.

One afternoon, another woman was admitted to our ICU. The emergency department was concerned she had a necrotizing soft tissue infection of her left leg. This diagnosis is not always straightforward, because the bacteria typically damage the layers of flesh underneath the skin, which makes their existence difficult to detect. Treatment needed to be initiated immediately. The treatment is to promptly cut away all of the flesh affected by the bacteria. We rushed her to the operating room and cut, cut, cut.

After surgery, we returned her to the burn unit to begin her recovery. Instead of getting better, though, she got worse. This can be a sign that we hadn't cut out all of the infection. It is not always easy to *get it all* the first time. Even the smallest bit of remaining infection can re-proliferate and kill the patient if not recognized and treated urgently. The woman became so sick that even moving her the slightest bit would cause her heart rate to skyrocket and her blood pressure to plummet to dangerous lows. This made it dangerous to move her back to the operating room to debride more tissue.

Given her tenuous state, the only remaining option was to amputate her leg to control the infection and save her life. But we could not agree on *how*. There are several ways to amputate a leg, typically all involving some variation of a saw. Because of how precarious the patient's clinical condition had become, however, it was agreed that the sudden loss of an extremity would push her already over-tasked body over the edge and kill her.

An older surgeon offered a solution I had never heard of before: *Cryoamputation,* or freezing off her leg using dry ice. Theoretically, this would result in a slower amputation process while still controlling the spread of infection and would be better tolerated by the patient.

The hospital didn't have dry ice, so we sent someone to the local supermarket to pick up several bags of it, as well as Styrofoam coolers. When they got back, we broke apart the Styrofoam coolers into sections, and used the sections to build an insulated barrier around the patient's leg. We packed dry ice around her leg, which was held in place by the Styrofoam pieces. We monitored her closely throughout the day, and she seemed to be tolerating our efforts—even getting better. We replenished the dry ice as needed, occasionally stealing glances at the now frost-bitten leg buried beneath. By evening the next day, her leg had been frozen enough that it could be easily removed without her body noticing. Miraculously, by the time my month in the burn unit had drawn to a close, she was still alive and stabilizing. Although I would not get to personally be there if she recovered and survived, I had every indication that she would.

During my rotation in the burn ICU, I worked six days a week, from five in the morning until whenever the work was done, which was typically sometime between seven and nine p.m. After rounding in the morning, we would operate for the rest of the day: Cut. Place hemostatic dressing. Remove hemostatic dressing. Burn. Place cadaver skin. Staple. Wrap in dressings. We did this day in and day out. Not only was the work tedious, but it was also physically demanding. I felt like the Greek legend Sisyphus: every morning I would begin pushing a boulder up a hill, only to have it roll back down overnight. Each day, I began rolling the boulder uphill again. Hard work aside, it was bearing witness to the endless misfortune of others that made the burn unit a nightmare.

This is how the entire rotation went; something horrific would happen, patients would be brought to the burn unit, and we would work tirelessly to take care of them. It was relentless work that never ended. The burn unit is like a machine that never gets turned off. It hums along, trying its best to undo nightmares. There was one upside, though: I realized I most definitely did not want to become a burn surgeon.

CHAPTER 11—Peanut Butter Pie

My rotation after the burn ICU was at a children's hospital. If the burn ICU was a nightmare, then the pediatric surgery was a house of horrors, which is unfortunate, because the holiday season was fast approaching. In an attempt to make the hospital more palatable to children, decorations began to pop up around the department. There were streamers, banners, lights, and trees, each decorated with a different theme and with presents piled high underneath. If I hadn't known any better, I might have thought I was at a theme park.

Our team of surgical residents was a motley one; we had all come from different hospitals. Our first-year intern, Darina, was a plastic surgery resident. Because plastic surgery has roots in general surgery, residents typically complete some of the same rotations we do.

Next on the team was Luis. I never found out what year resident he was. Over the next couple of months, I was able to partially piece together his story. He had done his intern year at one place, then done some general surgery residency at another, which he said was a "disaster," and was now here working as a 'research resident' in the pediatric surgery department. He would be one of the residents taking call for the entire year. This 'extra' time covering pediatric surgery made him very savvy and a great asset to our team.

Lastly was Dev. He was a third-year resident at a very well-known institution, who, like me, was there to gain mandatory exposure to pediatric surgery. Dev was by far the most serious of us all. I never saw him laugh once the entire time we worked together. Nevertheless, he worked hard and was easy to get along with. As I got to know him better, I found out that he had completed both medical school and a general surgery residency in India. The United States requires all practicing physicians to have completed a residency in either the United States or Canada. That is why Dev was doing general surgery residency for the second time. I couldn't imagine going through this hell twice.

The chief resident, our boss for the month, was the pediatric surgery fellow, Trent. I couldn't stand him, because he could be a real dick when he wanted to. He could get away with it, too, because he was also a really good surgeon. He had a tendency to rip one of us apart, then turn to the person next to him and be cheerful with them, as if nothing had just happened, leaving us standing in his wake beet faced and cheeks burning.

The horrors began on day one. Every morning the pediatric surgery attendings, fellows, residents, and nurse practitioners would gather and go through, or "run," the master list of all the patients. Mostly we discussed new patients that had been admitted overnight, as well as major updates on existing patients, so everyone would be on the same page at the beginning of every day. One of the new patients from the night before was a fifteen-year-old girl whose eyelids had been cut off.

Many people had tried to find out what happened, but the patient insisted that she had been walking home and that a dog had jumped on her and bitten them off. We reviewed images from the emergency department and realized that there were two major problems with her story. First, there were no other signs of a dog attack, no scratches or bite marks. Secondly, where her eyelids had been, was a clean cut, as if by a knife. There were no jagged edges suggesting they had been torn or ripped off like a dog would have done. Some sort of child abuse had definitely taken place. We did a quick search on our phones, and no one could identify any sort of cultural rituals in which eyelid removal was practiced. The girl was admitted to the hospital and the child welfare authorities were contacted. She would need her eyelids reconstructed by Darina and the plastic surgery department.

94

Taking call on the pediatric surgery service was similar to what I was used to, except instead of adults, our patient population now consisted of premature babies all the way to teenagers. Because there were four of us residents, we had to take call every fourth night, and more frequently if someone had been granted vacation.

I always felt like the hospital knew when a resident was starting their call shift, because at that precise moment, the trauma pager would start going off, nurses would barrage us with calls requesting various things for their patients, and the emergency department would hound us with new consults: "Hey, guess what, I've got another appy for you ..." Appy is shorthand for appendicitis. I don't know if there was something in the Phoenix water or what, but the number of kids needing appendectomies was endless.

At first, being pulled in so many different directions was overwhelming. And even after doing it for years, it could still be overwhelming. But no matter how late into the night it became, how tired or behind I got, I somehow always emerged the next day, alive.

Not only was Dev already a general surgeon in India, but he had started the rotation a few days prior to me. Combined with his relentlessly serious demeanor, I immediately trusted his judgement, and heeded his advice. The first day I was scheduled to take call, he was scheduled to work during the day, and he would be in the hospital with me until he went home in the evening and I remained overnight.

In the past, I had been accustomed to dividing work evenly among residents whenever possible. This early in residency, I was not yet comfortable asking other residents to do work, especially a resident I viewed as more advanced than me. So, I relied on the unspoken rule that we would *divide and conquer*. Dev had other plans. That day he told me that it would be my job to manage The List and see new consults, while he and Trent went to the operating room to operate. As surgical residents, all of us would rather operate.

I was caught off guard and couldn't muster the energy to argue. All morning, while I shuffled about the hospital doing scut work, discharging patients and seeing new consults, I grumbled to myself about how I had been tricked. Whenever the E.R. called me with a new consult, I would go and see the kid, diagnose them, and prepare them for surgery. Meanwhile, Dev stayed upstairs, tucked away in the O.R., performing the operations that I was serving up for him. As the day pressed on, I grew increasingly resentful of Dev and decided that I would confront him.

Once all of the operations were finished, around five p.m., Dev and I met up so that he could check out with me and leave. I was furious. In my head, I had been going over exactly what I was going to say to him. I didn't care if he was already a surgeon or how prestigious the hospital was that he was visiting from. He had taken advantage of me, and that was not OK.

We met in one of the small resident work rooms. He was sitting at a computer when I came in.

Before I could say anything, he looked up and said, "Hey, man, I want to show you something."

I figured he was going to show me something that he wanted me to take care of after he left. More work. I was about to lose my head and start yelling.

He continued, "Check it out, these five patients here," he said pointing, "I took care of all their discharge paperwork, printed their 'scripts, and put them in the charts. These two patients, I already got the parents to sign consents for surgery tomorrow, so you don't have to worry about that. And there is one more patient in the East Tower whose nurse didn't understand the orders you wrote this morning, so I went over and explained them to her."

Dev had stunned me for the second time that day. All day, he had been monitoring my progress on The List, and between O.R. cases he had been running around, silently helping me out. This was the opposite of what I had thought had been going on.

"I'm going to head out. See you tomorrow for rounds. When it's my turn to be on call, we'll switch, and you operate." And with that, he grabbed his backpack and left. After that, I was grateful we got to work together during those months. Although I tried several times, I never could get him to laugh, though.

Several weeks later, I was on call again. It had been a long day and a busy night so far. By two a.m., things seemed like they were quieting down, so I decided to try to get some sleep, something that rarely happens on call. I made my way through the bowels of the hospital, traveling through empty back hallways with exposed plumbing along the ceilings, eventually ending up at the call room. I checked the consult phone at every turn, suspicious that it wasn't ringing every couple of minutes. It was still quiet. Although the cramped, windowless call room appeared tidy, it smelled like dirty laundry. In the corner I saw the bed, although it was still made up, it was wrinkled and had clearly been used by someone, at some point. The room was like a motel; no one slept underneath the covers, they just lay on top for as long as they could before they got called to go do something. And that's exactly what I did.

Falling asleep while on call is always tough for me because I get anxious about missing an important call. What if something terrible happened, and it was my fault? I lay in bed and stared at the ceiling. Eventually, I fell asleep.

Sometime later the phone beeped like a crying baby demanding attention. Waking up after falling asleep on call is painful. My eyes shot open, but I couldn't see anything in the pitch-dark room. At first, I didn't know where I was, or what was going on. The phone was still shrieking, and I searched for it with my hand. My entire body hurt from head to toe. Finally, I found the phone and said the one word every caller seems to love to hear: "Surgery."

The voice on the other line was saying something about Tylenol.

"Fine. That's fine. Order it, put it under my name. Thanks," I said, and hung up. Normally nurses don't like receiving verbal orders over the phone, preferring the residents enter the orders into the computer themselves, but at night, if they're nice, sometimes they'll let you.

I almost fell back to sleep, but I was scared I would get called again and have to go through the pain of waking up all over again. I lay on the bed, my entire body aching. I contemplated my whole life, something else you only ever seem to do at night. Every person I knew on this planet was probably asleep. They got to sleep every single night, and they took it for granted. I was angry that I couldn't. I wished that I had chosen a different career. I hated my younger self for getting me into this. Not quite asleep and still half-awake, I felt delirious.

The phone rang again, this time it was a resident from the emergency department. The resident sounded frantic, something about a kid swallowing a battery. I told them I would be right there. While I made my way back through the bowels of the hospital to the emergency department, I thought about how overwhelmed the resident had sounded, and I wondered if emergency medicine was really the best career for them. Maybe they would be better suited for something with less emergencies, like wedding photography.

As I made my way downstairs, my pager went off. The E.D. resident had now upgraded the patient to a Level 1 trauma. This made me nervous, and I picked up my pace.

It was Saturday night, and I was on call with Trent. He had been riding me hard all day and I was utterly sick of him.

As I stepped into the trauma bay, I saw a boy about eighteen months old propped up on the gurney, crying, while people moved frantically around him.

"What's all the fuss?" I said to the red-faced emergency medicine resident who was darting around the room.

Hardly able to complete his sentences between breaths, I did manage to hear him spit out two words: "button battery."

"Did the patient swallow a button battery?" I asked, concerned.

Inhale, exhale, inhale, exhale, "YES!" he said finally, gesturing to X-ray images that were pulled up on the computer.

"Well, why didn't you say so?!" I said, studying the images which clearly showed what appeared to be a button battery lodged in the mid portion of the toddler's esophagus. I wondered if the emergency medicine resident would need medical attention, too.

The problem with button batteries—or the small flat batteries that usually go inside of watches—is that they can become lodged in the esophagus. While the esophagus tries to push the battery downwards into the stomach, the muscles can activate the battery by touching both the positive and negative sides simultaneously. If that happens, the battery can then erode through the esophagus and into the aorta which sits just behind the esophagus in the chest. That results in massive bleeding. If that happened, the baby would almost certainly bleed to death. And if *that* happened, everyone would get upset. This is why it was so important to remove the battery as quickly as possible, and to do that, the toddler had to be asleep.

By that point, Trent had shown up. He was also red in the face and looked stressed. Because the patient had been upgraded to Level 1, there was a decent-size crowd that had also shown up.

Here we go, I thought, waiting for him to begin berating me.

But for once, the thinly veiled insults didn't come. His wrath wasn't directed at me, but rather at the anesthesiologist, who hadn't shown up yet. Without the anesthesiologist, we couldn't put the kid to sleep and pull out the battery. His absence was like a bullfighter's red cape, temporarily distracting the angry bull, for now. I counted the seconds in my head until his absence would somehow become my fault. I braced myself for a verbal skewering.

Just then, the anesthesiologist strolled nonchalantly into the room, a fit older man I'd never seen before. He wore Poindexter-style glasses and an Air Force surgical cap. He was a complete juxtaposition against the chaos in the room. He exuded confidence and didn't hesitate when Trent started barking in his face.

"He swallowed a button battery, we have to take him up to the O.R., NOW!"

Cooly, he replied, "Okay," and continued as if it was business as usual. He was calm and nothing he said or did appeared rushed. I immediately liked him. If he had asked me to jump, I would have asked "How high?" If Trent, on the other hand, had asked me to jump, I probably would have argued with him for a little while and then, at the very last second, jumped barely high enough.

We quickly wheeled the tiny patient upstairs to the pre-operative area. The anesthesiologist began getting everything ready. He remained un-rushed but moved deliberately. He even paused for a moment to tell the bawling mother that everyone there that night with her son had kids and, they would treat her baby as if the child was one of their own. He put his hand on her shoulder, and for the first time since I had seen her, she stopped sobbing. I thought how cool he was. He made cucumbers look hot.

Meanwhile, Trent was growing impatient with the anesthesiologist. He paced around anxiously, his light skin turning darker and darker shades of red. He wouldn't *yell* at anyone. That wasn't his style; he was coyer than that. He inflicted pain with cleverly worded insults. But right now, he seemed too distracted to think of any.

Even though the anesthesiologist didn't appear to be rushing, he was moving efficiently. No time was being wasted. The young child was safe.

Hearing all the noise, Beverly, the head O.R. night nurse, joined us. A little on the heavy side, she was nearing the end of her career, and she was very loud herself. She was also fond of me and would often give me a hard time, but always in a friendly way. Maybe I reminded her of someone, a grandson perhaps. We also got along because of our unspoken dislike for Trent, although Beverly was much more open about it.

Beverly took in the unfolding scene, and then—as if she felt like she needed to add some commotion of her own—turned to me and (very loudly, as if nothing else was happening), started telling me about this peanut butter pie she had made. She said her and a couple of the other nighttime O.R. staff were just about to sit down and eat it when we *rudely* disrupted them by having to do this emergency case right now. I jokingly apologized for inconveniencing them, and I told her that I'd never had peanut butter pie before. I'd never even heard of it. That shocked her, and she told me I would have to try it after this whole mess was finished.

Out of the corner of my eye, I could see Trent growing even more furious as he watched Beverly chat with me. Beverly had always rubbed Trent the wrong way, mostly on purpose. Unlike me, however, Beverly wasn't bothered by Trent's scathing remarks. That only upset Trent even more. It was a small satisfaction for me to have them both there, because I could tell Trent resented the fact that Beverly and I got along so well.

The anesthesiologist was done with preparations. He picked up the toddler and carried the boy back to the operating room. Trent took off ahead of him, like a bull being released into an open pen for the first time. Once in the O.R., the anesthesiologist gently placed the kid onto the operating room table and began the process of sedating him.

Even in the operating room with the kid going to sleep, Trent was constantly moving around and fidgeting with things, as if he thought that constant movement was the only thing that could keep the baby alive.

The anesthesiologist placed a mask over the kid's mouth and gave him gases to put him to sleep. Once he was quiet and no longer moving, he took the mask off the child's face and used a laryngoscope to open the mouth before he inserted a tube that would provide him with oxygen while we removed the battery. During this, Trent had his back to the sleeping patient, and was anxiously fussing with the instruments on the scrub nurse's back table.

The anesthesiologist looked into the back of the toddler's mouth using the laryngoscope. Continuing to move with the same calm and confident manner, he reached over to his instrument tray and picked up a pair of Magill Forceps. They looked like an elongated pair of pliers, bent in the middle, and had wide tips. They were clearly designed for grabbing things. All of us except for Trent watched as he stuck the forceps into the back of the kid's mouth, moved them around a bit, and then, just like a magician, he pulled two coins out of the child: a penny and nickel.

"All done," he said.

Trent spun around and saw him standing there, holding the coins. It took him about half a second to figure out what had happened. There was no battery, and there never had been. The two coins had been lying on top of each other, lodged in the back of the boy's throat. When the emergency department resident had taken an X-ray, the two coins lying on top of each other had resembled a button battery. Trent turned even redder. The anesthesiologist had stolen his thunder. I could almost see smoke beginning to come out of his ears.

From across the room someone shouted, "1982!"

Then Beverly yelled, "1993!"

They were guessing the dates on the coins. We went around the room and then I joined in yelling, "2001!" Trent would make me pay for it later, but I didn't care; the coins were out, the kid was safe, and it had been a long day. It was okay to be happy for a moment. When it was his turn to guess, Trent of course, said nothing. He just stood there, steaming.

Once everyone had guessed, the anesthesiologist spread the coins out on his palms and read off the dates, "2018 and 2005." We had all been wrong, but we didn't care, we were having fun. I looked over at Trent, but he had already left. Then, the anesthesiologist woke the kid up and returned him and the coins to his parents, who were overjoyed. We sent them all home after reminding them that children aren't piggy banks.

The crowd of onlookers had thinned out by now. I knew where they had gone. I headed for the O.R. breakroom where I found Beverly, the anesthesiologist, and everyone else except for Trent. They were all sitting around, laughing and watching Beverly cut her peanut butter pie. I sat down with them, and Beverly cut me a slice. For a little while, we sat around and laughed and ate pie. I'd never had peanut butter pie before, and it was delicious. If I were to ever have it again, I don't know if it would taste as good. It was a nice escape, as brief as it was, but through the windows of the break room I could see that the sun was beginning to rise. A moment later my pager started beeping. Our brief late-night hiatus from the rigors of healthcare had come to a screeching halt. Time to start rounding, time to get back to work.

Just like with burn surgery, though, I knew that pediatric surgery was not for me.

CHAPTER 12—10,000 Hours

It has been said that it takes 10,000 hours of doing something to become an expert. Let's do some basic math. Residency was five years long. There are fifty-two weeks in a year, but let's say I only worked forty-eight of them. That's 240 weeks. Furthermore, let's round down and say that I only worked sixty to seventy hours per week. This means that by the end of residency, I would have accumulated between 14,400 and 16,800 work hours. That's more than enough to be considered an expert. If I truly did work the maximum eighty hours per week, or more, which is entirely possible, then by these calculations, I would have worked 19,200+ hours. Nearly double the number needed to be considered an expert.

At first, being in the hospital all hours of the day and night was fun and exciting. But by the end of my second year, 100 weeks into residency, the fatigue began to catch up, and it had become a chore to go to work. I began to resent being a resident. Each morning I spent longer and longer in my car outside of the hospital, contemplating going back home. I had to talk myself into going to work. I had lost my enthusiasm for surgery. Medicine in general was getting boring. Patients' constant complaints of pain and hunger became annoying. Even my hobbies were losing their appeal.

One morning, I was doing rounds and went into a sleeping patient's room. He had broken most of his bones, and when he was awake, he was in constant pain. As I watched him sleep, I remember wishing that I could trade places with him, just so that I could lie in bed and sleep. I didn't know it at the time, but this was the beginning of burnout.

I didn't share how I felt with anyone. Among family and friends, I was a new hot shot doctor well on my way to becoming a great surgeon. I did not want to disappoint them. At times, even if I did start to bring it up, they wouldn't understand, saying things like "it's just a phase." To attending surgeons, I was already a part of the wimpy generation of residents that were protected by the *eighty-hour work week* rule—a work limit established in 2008. Anything I mentioned about how I felt would only come off as a complaining. Among peers, I wanted to be seen as tough, one of them. I couldn't risk losing their acceptance. Because none of us ever talked about it, I didn't know if anyone else felt the same way. Although I was constantly surrounded by people—some of whom might have been experiencing the same burnout as I was—I felt isolated, and I wanted out.

We never talked about our internal struggles or how we felt, so I was surprised when one of my co-residents, Jeff, told me he was quitting at the end of our second year. Initially, I thought he was being sarcastic, or overreacting. After all, we had all worked so hard to get here, how could he just give it all up like that?

The more we talked about it, the more I realized how serious he was. Jeff had already made arrangements to join another residency program, in family medicine. Not only would he be free from the brutal hours of surgery residency, he would also no longer have to work overnight, weekends, and, because family medicine is only a three-year residency, he would graduate and become an attending physician before me! When I thought about how much free time and sleep he would soon get, I became envious of his resolve.

That Friday, Jeff told our residency program director, Dr. Moore, of his plans. Bursting with curiosity, I met up with him afterward to find out how it had gone.

"How'd it go? Did she tell you to get back to work?" I said, half-jokingly.

"Not quite. She gave me the weekend off and told me to think about it. Not to do anything rash," came his calm response.

"Do you think you'll change your mind?"

"Not a chance. My wife and I have been talking about this for a while," he replied with conviction.

I wondered to myself if being vulnerable with his wife about how much he hated surgical residency had changed what she thought of him. Did she now think that she had married a quitter? Maybe he was so burned out he no longer cared what she thought? I had just started a new relationship, and I was far from being married. Being vulnerable and discussing quitting residency was nowhere near the list of things to talk about with a new girlfriend. Now I was jealous of Jeff for another reason. I worked over the weekend and anxiously awaited seeing Jeff on Monday.

"Well?" I said, when I finally caught up with him.

He smiled, knowing exactly what I was referring to. "I did it. I told her I am for sure out."

"Seriously?" I asked, still skeptical.

"Yup. I'm going to finish out this year and that's it. Since I'm leaving surgery, the remainder of my schedule will be adjusted so that I no longer have go into the O.R. and operate. I'll just be doing patient care on the wards for the rest of the time."

Fumbling for what to say next, "Do you think you'll regret it?"

He chuckled again, "No way. I'm really looking forward to it, man. If you're unhappy, I really encourage you to think about doing it too."

This last part gave me pause. Why did he say that? Did he know I was unhappy? Had I been acting differently? Would others think I might want to quit, too? Even though it was true, I didn't want people to know it.

I thought about what Jeff had done and wondered if I should do the same. If I *could* do the same. Jeff had clearly thought this through very carefully, going as far as to make arrangements for a different residency program. I had not. Quitting to me was still a fantasy, something I thought about in the middle of the night while I was awake on call when I'd rather be sleeping. Unlike Jeff, I didn't have a plan. And also, unlike Jeff, who had clearly discussed how he felt with his wife and had her full support, I hadn't discussed how I felt with anyone. I had just begun dating my girlfriend, and I didn't want to scare her off by giving her the impression that I was a quitter. Furthermore, if I up and quit, it would be a shock to everyone who had always known me as a surgery fanatic. How would I explain my change of heart to them?

Would they understand? These questions swirled around my mind. I was too busy to sit down and thoroughly consider each one—or at least, that was the excuse I gave myself. Suddenly, quitting felt like more work than not, so, as Jeff moved on and left the program, I put any plans I had to quit on the back burner for the time being and kept going.

Like almost all careers, a career in medicine comes with occupational health risks. We are exposed to radiation from X-ray machines. We're exposed to potentially deadly diseases from patients and needle sticks, or smoke inhalation from cautery in the operating room. We develop neck and back issues from decades of hunching over patients. Some—many, even—self-medicate as a way of coping with the stresses of work and some develop substance abuse issues. Of this sub-group, many develop opioid addiction from having easy access to them (this issue is most pronounced in the field of anesthesiology). And for reasons that aren't entirely clear, we are at an increased risk of suicide.

During my third year of residency, physician burnout and well-being had become a hot topic within the medical community. There had been a growing amount of media attention devoted to rising physician and resident suicide rates in the US.

Multiple sources state that approximately 300 physicians commit suicide annually. To put that into perspective, that is as if two to three entire graduating classes of medical students were to commit suicide each year. The exact reasons for why this happens is unclear, but for the first time, people were now considering that burnout could be a major contributing factor. The Accreditation Council for Graduate Medical Education (AGCME) mandated that hospitals with residency programs institute some sort of wellness initiative.

Hospitals across the country began adopting physician wellness campaigns. For the most part, these early campaigns consisted mostly of recommendations to practice yoga at lunch or go on a relaxing walk. These campaigns were misinformed. Did anyone really think that asking physicians to give up their precious few minutes to eat lunch and do yoga somewhere in the hospital was going to convince a suicidal doctor to re-consider? Another possibility is that these campaigns were simply a means of acknowledging the problem until a durable solution could be arrived at. I will point out that, among all of the wellness discussions that took place, decreasing physician work hours was never once considered.

At my hospital, wellness committees were formed. Two residents from each specialty were selected to act as resident representatives. I was chosen to be one of them. Our first resident wellness committee meeting took place on a Wednesday afternoon. A meeting room had been rearranged so that all of the tables were pushed against the walls and the chairs placed in a circle facing each other. In the middle of the circle sat a psychologist.

After a lengthy introduction in which we were vigorously assured of the psychologist's credentials, we launched into the classic "Stand up, introduce yourself, and tell us something fun about you!" icebreaker.

While residents popped up from their chairs like groundhogs to introduce themselves, I scanned the room taking note of which other residents were being held hostage with me; family medicine ... internal medicine ... pain and rehabilitation medicine ... and ... dermatology?! "What was dermatology doing here? *What could possibly be making dermatology residents burn out?* I wondered.

Once the introductions were out of the way, we were then asked to each share a traumatic experience which we had been faced with in residency. Everyone's stories were similar: a patient they had been caring for a long time continued to get sicker and sicker; eventually the patient needed to be transferred to the intensive care unit; and then they died.

Dermatology residents worked exclusively in the outpatient clinic setting. Unable to relate to this common theme, one of them spoke up, eager to share one of her traumatic experiences.

She jumped to her feet and said, "Well, this one time I was in clinic, and there was this patient who was being very difficult. I had to stay until five-thirty p.m. trying to help him."

Looking around the room at our blank faces, she quickly added, "Clinic normally closes at four-thirty p.m.! I had to stay an hour late; it really messed up my afternoon."

The room was silent. Even the psychologist struggled to find words to say. I was stunned that she had felt this story was appropriate to tell, after how serious everyone else's stories had been.

Eventually, it became my turn to share. Until that moment, I had not felt like participating and I'd planned to tell a similar story as everyone else. But now I was a little bit irritated by the dermatology resident's choice of personal trauma and decided to tell a particularly gut-wrenching tale instead.

I stood up. "I was on call the other night. Around two in the morning I got paged that a level 1 trauma was coming in. Then another page, and another page, and another page. Four level 1 traumas all coming at once." I looked around the room, everyone's eyes were focused on me. "At first, I thought it was a mistake, that the dispatcher hit the button too many times or something. But when I got down to the E.R. the paramedics were already streaming in, bringing patient after patient. As it turned out, two SUV's full of high school kids were street racing just down the street from here, and they both crashed. Several kids died on the scene. The medics scooped up the ones that weren't dead and rushed them to us. Myself and the attending surgeon who were on call that night quickly went from bed to bed quickly triaging each of the kids. We were able to save two of them, but two more died." I abruptly sat back down, finished.

The room was silent again. I immediately regretted what I had done. I had used what had been a tragedy for several families as ammunition to retaliate against the dermatology resident's lame story. Or maybe I hadn't realized how badly I had needed to talk about it. I'm not sure.

"How did you deal with that?" the psychologist asked.

"I just went back to work. To be honest, I hadn't even thought about it again until just now."

Eventually we moved on, the discussion moving on to how being on call could be made better for residents. By now, you may have noticed that I don't like being on call. No one does. Sleep deprivation is physically and mentally exhausting. There's a reason it's used as a form of illegal torture.

Before anyone could say anything, the dermatology resident was back on her feet already obnoxiously offering her perspective.

"I remember one night when I was on call being so stressed out, and then someone showed me the hospital had Pacman. I played it and felt a whole lot better."

Initially, I thought she was making a bad joke. But the psychologist was intrigued. Cluelessly, she asked the dermatology resident at which hospital she took call.

Sitting back down, she leaned back in her chair distractedly examining her fingernails, she replied, "Dermatology doesn't actually take any call. I just thought it was a nice idea."

Astounded, I thought to myself, *If only the solution were as simple as that.*

Since this time, I am happy to report that physician burnout has continued to gain awareness. Some refer to it as "healing the healer" or "caring for the caregiver." Slowly, but surely, a cultural shift is taking place.

As I left that meeting, I considered physician burnout and wellness to be a joke. Since then, it has become an issue that is near and dear to my heart. During my five years as a resident, two attending surgeons that I worked with and admired, passed away from suicide. And unbeknownst to me at the time, I was burning out.

CHAPTER 13—Communication is Key

Speaking with patients is an art. Explaining complicated medical topics can be tricky. It's not always easy to bridge the gap between what patients understand and what I understand after years of medical training. On top of that, everyone communicates a little bit differently. Some patients want to know everything, others want to know as little as possible, some nod their head as if they understand what I am saying (when in fact they don't). Meanwhile, other patients interrupt me so frequently that I forget what I was trying to say in the first place.

The art, which I was attempting to master, was figuring out how to effectively communicate with the patient in front of me, knowing little about them, other than their medical history.

A wise surgeon once told me a story that I have carried with me since. "There was a study in which the same doctor went into a room with different patients," he told me, "and it was timed how much time he spent with each patient. Afterward, the patients were asked to estimate how much time the doctor had spent with them. The doctor spent less than two minutes with every patient, but the patients in which he did the three things with, all estimated that he had spent five minutes with them, more than double as long as he actually had! Can you guess what those three things are?"

I had no idea. No one had ever told me about such a study before. I guessed things like, "Always having an answer for their questions," and "acting in a professional manner."

"Wrong," he said, smiling. "The three things are," he continued, counting out each with his fingers, "one, you must sit down. If you're in a room with no stool, sit on the edge of their bed. You have to be eye level with them. Two, touch the patient, even if there is no medically necessary reason to. For example, if a patient comes to you complaining of a headache, touch their head, pretend you are examining it, but touch it. There is an incredible power in human touch. And lastly, talk about at least one thing other than what is wrong with them. It's so easy to get caught up discussing all of the symptoms associated with someone's abdominal pain, but never forget that patients aren't their disease. They are real people with lives outside their disease, just like you and I, and they want to be treated as such. If someone has on a baseball cap, I'll ask them if it's their favorite team. You get the idea."

I did get the idea. Since that day, his words have remained seared into my brain. From then on, I made an effort to try to do those three things each time I interacted with a patient, hoping soon it would become automatic.

In residency, one afternoon per week, we ran a clinic. It was located a few blocks from the hospital in what appeared to be an old house that had been converted to a doctors' office. The office wasn't owned by any doctor in particular but was instead shared amongst several specialties that all used the building for their weekly clinics. Most frequent of which was the family medicine doctors.

The clinic had been set up to help serve patients without insurance who had no other access to healthcare. This created for us a steady stream of patients who had surgical issues that spanned the gamut.

I know what you are thinking: that it's unjustified to "practice" and "learn" how to do surgery on people who can't afford "a real doctor." But this was far from that. Our clinic, and the operations we performed, were all carefully monitored, and I promise you, that each and every patient received quality care.

For all intents and purposes, our clinic functioned as a shortcut to get patients without insurance to bypass the hospital's "facility fee" and get them into the hospital where they could receive surgery without a massive bill.

It works like this: the majority of the expenses associated with surgery don't come from the surgeon or the anesthesiologist. They come from the hospital charging a "facility fee" (sometimes disguised under a different name). The facility fee can range from a thousand dollars to hundreds of thousands of dollars. Ostensibly, this fee is meant to cover the cost the hospital incurs for a given surgery; maintaining a working operating room, paying the electricity bill to keep the lights on, keeping the operating room clean, stocking it with supplies, paying nurses, etc. Longer, more complex surgeries, cost more, and they make more money for the hospital.

Unfortunately, for patients looking to shop around, the fee is impossible to predict ahead of time since the rates that hospitals charge are not standardized and vary from hospital to hospital and patient to patient. If someone doesn't have insurance, or their insurance provider declines to pay, then the unlucky patient is left to foot the enormous bill. Recently, hospitals have come under public and government scrutiny in response to allegations that for some patients this fee gets over-inflated, ballooning up to tens of thousands of dollars more than other patients paid for the same operation at the same hospital. At the end of the day, hospitals (non-profit or for-profit alike) are businesses.

Our clinic was a hospital charity. The hospital would allow us to operate on patients who came through our clinic, without being charged a facility fee (or a greatly reduced one). We also had anesthesiologists on board who would help us with our cases, pro-bono, and our attending surgeons of course, didn't send a bill either. As a result, the clinic was slightly underfunded. This is where we residents fit in. Although we had staff that was friendly and eager to help, additional help from the residents was needed to bring all of the pieces together. And of course, it was a valuable learning experience. Furthermore, our patients were always grateful for our time (which was not always the case elsewhere), and we enjoyed treating them.

One day, my chief resident Jeremy and I were seeing a twenty-six-year-old woman for a follow-up visit. She had come to our clinic the week before with a complaint of swelling around the front of her neck. When we examined her, we had discovered that her thyroid gland was asymmetrically enlarged, indicating that there was a mass inside of it: a tumor. During her last visit, we had biopsied the mass so that the pathologist could analyze and identify which type of tumor it was. Today we were seeing her in the clinic to discuss with her the results of the biopsy, which confirmed the mass was indeed cancer.

We stood in the hallway and knocked on the door before we entered the room. The young woman was sitting alone on the exam table, playing on her phone. She didn't look very concerned. Jeremy and I sat down across from her—him on the doctor stool and me on a chair off to the side. The plan was for him to do most of the talking—to show me how it was done—while I observed.

Jeremey started by asking the woman, "Tell me what you understand so far about what is going on." This allows the doctor to gauge the patient's understanding so that everyone can start on the same page.

"I have something in my thyroid. Last week you took a little piece of it to help figure out what it is, and today you're going to have the results."

What she said was correct, but what she didn't say was that she understood there was a chance it could be cancer.

As soon as she was done speaking, Jeremy immediately began to reply. I suspected he was nervous, and instead of listening to what she was saying, he had probably been mentally rehearsing what he was going to say.

"So, the biopsy came back with papillary thyroid carcinoma," he said, and without pausing to explain what this meant, he continued. "It looks like it's about four centimeters in its largest dimension. That's just a little bit too big to only take half of the thyroid gland out, so we will recommend taking the whole thing out."

Finally, he paused. She sat there, silently staring at him, so he continued, "There are some risks associated with the procedure. Like with any procedure, there is a risk of bleeding, infection, and damage to surrounding structures. Specifically in this case, there is a risk of damaging the recurrent laryngeal nerve and a branch of the recurrent laryngeal nerve called the superior recurrent laryngeal nerve ..." He continued to elaborate on the risks of surgery.

The patient remained frozen, staring at him, and he continued to describe to her the technical details of the surgery. Everything he was saying was correct, but to me, he sounded more like he was giving a lecture on thyroid surgery rather than speaking to a patient.

Then, suddenly, interrupting Jeremy's description of how her parathyroid glands would be protected during surgery, she frantically burst out, "I HAVE CANCER?!"

Jeremy stopped talking. He seemed confused and unsure of what to say next. He glanced over at me, bewildered. In his mind, when he had told her she had papillary thyroid carcinoma, he had already established that she had cancer.

Confused about where he had gone wrong, he tried, "Um, yes. You have cancer in your thyroid gland."

Upon hearing this, she burst into tears.

Desperately, he added, "It's very treatable, though!" But it had no effect. She continued to sob. He looked at me and shrugged obliviously.

Having witnessed the entire interaction, it was clear to me what had gone wrong. But in that moment, not wanting to make him feel any worse, I shrugged my shoulders back at him.

Eventually, she stopped crying, and we were able to start over, explain to her what papillary thyroid carcinoma is—a very slow growing tumor with an exceptionally high survival rate—and discuss different treatment options with her.

By the time we had finished, she understood exactly what was going on and what needed to be done next. A few weeks later, we performed surgery without any issues, and she did fine.

Experiences like this are important, underscoring the need to communicate effectively. I've seen many different physicians communicate with patients in many different ways. I've seen physicians go back and forth, answering the barrage of questions nervous patients ask, effortlessly tossing back answers to everything thrown at them. I've watched others sit with their patients, and in a soothing voice, tell them next to nothing about their diagnosis or the surgery required. I've even seen others confidently steamroll over everything their patient says, shake their hand, and leave.

Figuring out how to communicate effectively with patients is part of why medicine is sometimes referred to as an art. Unsurprisingly, I've found that older physicians tend to be better at reading patients and making these judgement calls. Although there are plenty of articles written on the topic of effective communication, like leadership, it is best learned through experience.

CHAPTER 14—Friday Night Lights

After a busy Friday, I had completed my usual routine of driving to the hospital and debating whether or not I should go home, I had taken sign-out from Kyle, pre-rounded on the patients, run The List with the chief, assisted on five operations, and in between each, seen seven new consults. But my day was only half over. I was slated to be on call that night and I was already physically exhausted from running around the hospital and mentally exhausted from keeping track of every patient. To top things off, on Fridays, the hospital was full of "Thank God It's Friday" chatter from weekday warriors who are looking forward to having their weekend free. Not me. I was only halfway through my "shift," and I was ready to collapse.

Around four-thirty p.m., I was standing in the O.R., scrubbed in. Justin Beiber's remix of *Despacito* was playing overhead on the speakers. We were about to repair a ventral hernia on a patient named Kevin, a healthy young man in his thirties. It was our last scheduled surgery of the day. A ventral hernia is a weakness in the abdominal wall that causes a bulge. It's most common in obese patients. For some this bulge can be painful, others find it disfiguring. For us, the surgery is routine.

The scrub tech handed me the scalpel and I loudly announced "Incision!" as I slid the belly of the scalpel across the patient's abdomen, making the first cut.

"Why so big!?" Dr. Yang, the attending surgeon, was screaming at me from across the table. "It's a tiny hernia! What has this patient ever done to you?!"

"Sorry," I mumbled, trying to maintain my focus. It was late in the afternoon, and I knew he was eager for me to make a mistake so that he would have an excuse to take the operation from me, finish it quickly, and go home. I was determined to not let that happen.

"Scalpel back!" I said loudly as I handed the scalpel back to the scrub tech, alerting her so that she would not cut herself.

Without me having to ask, she handed me the Bovie, the lightsaber of surgery. Carefully, so as not to irritate Dr. Yang further, I meticulously dissected each layer of the patient's abdominal wall, the Bovie vaporizing the tissue as I did. Each swipe of the instrument took us closer and closer to the patient's insides.

"Pull, please," I said to Dr. Yang as my incision grew deeper.

I heard a derisive huff from underneath Dr. Yang's mask. He had been hoping I would forget this step and struggle, which would have provided him with the perfect excuse to take over the operation. If I was still a first- or second- year, then maybe this would have happened, but I was a third-year now.

He curled his fingers into the edge of my incision on his side of the table gently retracting it toward himself. With my right hand, I did the same on my side, continuing to dissect with the Bovie in my left hand.

"Careful!" came Dr. Yang's voice as I approached the final layer of the abdominal wall, the only remaining barrier between us and the inside of the patient's abdomen. If I wasn't careful and I went too fast, I could damage the patient's intestines or another one of his vulnerable organs.

"Not today," I murmured to myself. "Okay, I'm going to get us in now," I said, signaling to Dr. Yang that I was going to incise the final layer, granting us access to the inside of the patient's abdomen.

"Okay, just don't damage the bowel or I'll kill you," he retorted. I knew he was joking. At least partially.

I made the final incision and was immediately met with a rush of yellow fluid that burst from the patient's abdomen, spilling over the sides of the drapes onto us.

"What the fuck did you do?!" Dr. Yang shouted at me as he slapped my hands away from the patient and replaced them with his own.

117

Stunned, I thought to myself, *What did I do?* Fearing the worst, that I had just damaged our patient, I stood frozen, as Dr. Yang inserted a suction catheter into the wound, quickly removing the fluid so that he could see what was underneath.

I watched as over six liters of straw-colored fluid were suctioned out of the patient. I could feel my toes starting to become damp as the fluid that had spilled onto us soaked into my socks.

"Fuck! It's cancer! Fuck!" Dr. Yang was shouting as he looked through the incision into the patient's abdomen. "Fuck!"

I was still frozen in place, trying to figure out what had just happened.

"Get the retractor in here! Come on, let's go! Help me out, Ryan, I can't fucking see!" he was screaming.

Hastily, the scrub tech and I worked to assemble the large metal retractor which consisted of a giant oval shaped ring with several smaller arms designed to hold open the patient's abdomen, which freed up our hands to work inside. Meanwhile, I thought to myself, *Cancer ...? Not possible. He's overreacting. He always overreacts. This is a healthy thirty-year-old guy."*

Once we had the retractor in place Dr. Yang shouted, "There! Right there!" And pointed with the tip of his metal instrument.

I looked but didn't see anything. "Where?" I asked, cautiously.

"Right there, goddamnit! Are you even paying attention!" he said, grabbing my hand and thrusting it into the patient's abdomen, rubbing my fingertips against something rough.

Sure enough, I felt the rubbery rough texture that had become all too familiar to me during residency. He was right. It was cancer. I moved my hand and squinted. All over the inside of the patient's abdomen were coarse little bumps that looked like tiny mushrooms. The magnitude of the disease meant that it was metastatic. It was these tiny tumors that had generated the fluid that had filled the patient's abdomen. The patient had been misdiagnosed. He didn't have a hernia because he had gained weight and become obese; he had a hernia because his abdomen had been filling up with fluid.

"Biopsy it," Dr. Yang was saying to me. Then, to the O.R. nurse, he

118

demanded, "Call the pathologist. Tell him to come in now."

I asked for the scalpel back and used it to cut away a few of the small bumps. I placed them in a small plastic cup to be taken immediately to the pathology lab. The pathologist had no doubt gone home for the weekend and would be annoyed at having to come back to examine this specimen under the microscope. It's very uncommon for the pathologist on-call to have to return to the hospital. There are very few diagnostic conundrums that require an urgent consultation. This, however, was one of them. We needed to know exactly what we were dealing with in order to proceed correctly.

The nurse rushed out of the room with the specimen, leaving us standing in the O.R. We waited. Dr. Yang stood with his arms folded, looking at the ground and tapping his foot. We discussed our options. We were confident this was cancer but needed the pathologist to examine it under his microscope and officially confirm. The surgery had changed. We were no longer performing a routine hernia surgery, but instead diagnosing someone with cancer. *Advanced* cancer.

Suddenly aware of the gravity of what was happening, the O.R. staff became quiet. Just a few minutes earlier, everyone had been discussing their weekend plans. The entire tone had changed. After what felt like hours, the phone rang. The O.R. nurse ran over, answered it and placed it on speaker phone.

"Hello? It's Rob, can you hear me?" the pathologist's voice echoed through the room.

"Yeah, we can hear you! What the fuck is it!?" Dr. Yang yelled at the phone from across the room.

"Well ... it's hard to say for sure. I'm seeing a lot of atypia, distorted nuclei, dysplasia ..." his voice trailed off.

"Is it cancer?!" Dr. Yang was screaming again.

"Well, uh, yeah, it's definitely cancer. I just don't know what type yet."

"I knew it. Thanks." Then more quietly to the nurse, "hang up the phone." Then, Dr. Yang spoke to me across the sleeping patient on the operating room table. "Close him." And with that, he pulled off his surgical gown.

"What about the hernia?" I asked.

"Don't fix it. The fluid will re-accumulate in a few days, and it will only come back. He has other more important things to worry about now. Just close him."

Stunned by these unexpected findings, I worked quietly as I closed each layer of the incision that I had worked so carefully to create.

Despising the silence, I asked, "Where do you think it came from?"

"I have no idea," Dr. Yang replied, sitting on a stool pensively while I worked. "We won't know until the final pathology stains come back. And even then, we still may not know."

I didn't bother bringing up prognosis. There was nothing to discuss. We both knew it was bad. The fact that the cancer was studded all over each surface of his abdomen meant that it was by definition metastatic. Stage 4. The highest of all the cancer stages. I glanced over the surgical drapes at the patient's face, noting again how young he was. We were nearly the same age. My entire life had been meticulously structured around planning for the future. In another year, it was unlikely this patient would still be alive.

After I finished closing the patient's abdomen, I tore off my surgical gown and picked up the patient's medical chart. I rifled through the papers searching for a listed emergency contact. I wanted to call someone close to him and let them know how he was doing. He would be too drowsy after waking up from anesthesia to understand. My heart dropped, because no emergency contact had been listed. The patient was here completely alone. There was no one else in the world for me to call and update on how he was doing. I would later find out that he had immigrated to the US by himself, leaving his family behind, so that he could get a job and send money back to them.

I stopped by the cafeteria and discovered they were serving leftover meatloaf from lunch. I was elated. I missed lunch earlier and didn't know it was meatloaf day. Hospital meatloaf can be contentious: you either hated it or loved it. I loved it. I stacked a few pieces onto my plate, as well as some overcooked vegetables, and made my way down the hall to the resident work room.

I plopped down on the couch in the resident work room and placed my food on the couch next to me. I avoided putting my food on the coffee table because I've seen other residents put their feet on it too many times. My socks were still squishy with my prior patient's abdominal fluid, and everyone else whose feet have rested on that table has been through a similar adventure.

"You need a list?" Kyle asked, turning away from the bank of computers and facing me.

I pulled my list from the morning out of my pocket and looked at it. It was covered in tiny, barely legible, writing. The paper contained not only the notes I took in the morning, but also notes that I'd been writing to myself throughout the day about each patient. Despite the fact that I had worked tirelessly throughout the day trying to keep my list up to date, it was now outdated. Medicine moves fast. Patients who were on my list have since been discharged from the hospital, and new ones who aren't on it have been admitted.

"Yeah, print me one, will you?" I replied, as I sliced off a piece of meatloaf and shoved it into my mouth.

The printer hummed to life in the corner of the room. "I can't believe you're eating that!" Kyle said, watching me.

I shrugged, my mouth too full to reply.

Kyle got up and pulled the new list out of the printer. It was four pages long. While I ate, he updated me on each patient: why they were in the hospital, what surgery they'd had, or were going to have, what diet they were allowed, and most importantly, what (if any) emergency situation might arise for them overnight.

I listened carefully and jotted down a few notes between bites. Once Kyle and the rest of the residents went home, I would be responsible for troubleshooting any issues that arose throughout the night, even answering questions from their nurses—even though I hadn't met most of the patients. The sign-out Kyle gave me would be critical to avoiding medical errors. Despite the fact that he gave me a comprehensive sign-out, it's inevitable that I'd be dealing with issues that he hadn't been able to foresee. It would be up to me to use my medical judgement in the middle of the night to avoid a catastrophe.

Half an hour later, Kyle waved goodbye over his shoulder as he walked out the door. I'd finished eating and tilted my head back on the couch. I closed my eyes, bracing for what I anticipated would be a long night. I briefly drifted off before the trauma pager woke me with its incessant beeping. I groaned and glanced down at the tiny screen: **Level 1 Trauma Activation. ETA *6 minutes by ground.*** Level 1 trauma activations are the highest level of activation, reserved for only the sickest and most damaged patients. I rubbed the sleep from my eyes and stood up. "Game time."

Although I had only drifted off for ten minutes, I felt refreshed. I strolled into the emergency department and headed over to the trauma bay, where people had started to gather and prepare for the arrival of our trauma patient. I made my way inside, leaned against a counter, and waited. The trauma bay is a room in the emergency department that is larger than a typical patient room and resembles a small operating room, complete with a bed in the middle and a surgical light that hangs overhead.

Just like with code blues, the team that assembles is a crowd. It filled the large trauma bay and spilled out into the hall. Each member of the team had a designated role. Aside from myself, the team consisted of nurses, laboratory technicians, a pharmacist, respiratory therapists, X-ray technicians, security guards, an emergency room physician, nursing and medical students, as well as the occasional curious hospital employee who just happened to be passing by.

There was one more person that also showed up: the captain of the ship, the conductor of the orchestra, the attending trauma surgeon. On that night, it was Dr. Smith, a young surgeon with wire-rimmed glasses who had only finished his training five years ago. Because I was still a resident, my role would be that of co-pilot to Dr. Smith.

The large crowd of people could sometimes make trauma surgery feel like a spectator sport. Every time the trauma surgeon makes a decision, gives an instruction, or performs a procedure, it happens in front of the crowd.

The crowd at the trauma bay liked working on trauma. They'd seen many trauma activations before. And if they didn't agree with how things were unfolding, they would be vocal about it. Amid all this chaos, it was the trauma surgeon's responsibility to filter out the noise and perform. Just like the hospital meatloaf, this added pressure was not for everyone. Some hated it, but others, like me, loved it.

Once the trauma patient arrived, the team would descend on him, swarming around like ants who just discovered a piece of leftover bread. Everyone would perform their unique role, doing everything they were capable of doing to prevent a total stranger from dying. This was the trauma center's big show, a symphony of well-choreographed chaos. Each person played their role like an instrument while the trauma surgeon conducted the show. To an outsider, it looked a mob scene, but to an experienced eye, it was harmonious.

Still leaning on the counter, I shouted across the room to the charge nurse, "What do we have coming?"

"Sixteen-year-old boy. Coming from a high school football game down the road. Stable vitals but he's unconscious," she shouted back.

Boring, I thought. This sort of thing happened all the time, and they nearly never required surgery. Often, during a game, a kid gets hit and briefly loses consciousness. Out of an abundance of caution, someone calls an ambulance. Typically, by the time the patient arrives they have regained consciousness and are fine. We diagnose them with a concussion, and they go home. It's what football coaches sometimes refer to as a "bell ringer," because the player got their bell rung.

While we waited for the ambulance to arrive, the room buzzed with small talk. It's impossible to get this many people together in one place and expect them to wait in silence.

About five minutes later, someone shouted down the hallway, "They're here! They're here!"

We quieted down and watched as the paramedics wheeled the patient into the trauma bay. It was immediately clear that something wasn't right. On the stretcher was a motionless teenager still wearing his football jersey. He wasn't awake like I'd been expecting. This was not typical.

We quickly transferred him to the trauma bay bed and began to assess him. Someone mentioned that his name was Antonio. I ground my knuckles into his breastbone, a maneuver called a *sternal rub*, which is meant to inflict a great deal of pain without causing harm. Typically, this is enough to elicit some sort of response from patients who are unconscious. This time though, there was nothing. He wasn't moving at all. This was alarming. I pulled up his eyelids and looked at his eyes. Both of his pupils were dilated and didn't constrict when exposed to the bright light of the trauma bay. Another alarming finding. This is what is known as *blown pupils*, and it was indicative of a severe brain injury.

Dr. Smith instructed the emergency medicine physician to insert a breathing tube. As soon as he finished, I shouted to the room, "Give him 100 grams of mannitol and let's go! We need to get in the CT scanner now and get a look at what's going on inside his head!"

The mannitol would help temporarily decrease the swelling in his brain while we got more information from the CT scan to determine the best next course of action. I needed to see his brain. If we were early enough, we could potentially still intervene and save him.

As the nurses rushed the patient from the trauma bay down the short hallway to the CT scanner, I turned to the paramedics and asked them what had happened. Realizing the seriousness of the situation, they now appeared a little bit shaken.

"When we got there, we were told that he had been tackled and went unconscious, then had a brief seizure on the field."

"Any history of seizure disorder?" I asked them.

"I don't think so. Both of his parents were there watching the game and we were only able to talk to them briefly. They told us he has never had a seizure before."

"How big was the kid that hit him?" I asked, trying to get a sense of *exactly* what had happened.

"About the same size as him, but we were told it was a helmet-to-helmet hit and the patient's helmet came off. Do you think he'll be okay?"

"I don't know," I said, ducking into the room with the CT scanner, leaving them in the hall.

We all stood quietly, holding our breath, waiting for the CT technician to start the scan. There was a low-pitched mechanical whirring sound as the machine sprang to life, and then slowly, images of the patient's brain began to appear on the screen.

There was a collective groan. We all recognized the image on the screen which showed the patient's brain pushed to the side of his skull by a large white mass that, ironically, was shaped like a football. This is the classic presentation of an *epidural hematoma*, a type of intracranial hemorrhage. It occurs when an artery on the inside of the skull bleeds. Like blood coming out of a firehose, it can bleed with such force that it crushes the soft brain, causing irreversible damage and sometimes, death. Our only hope now was to cut open the side of his skull and attempt to stop the bleeding. We wouldn't be able to reverse whatever damage had already been done, but maybe we could prevent further damage.

I called the on-call neurosurgeon, Dr. Rashid, right away and described to him what we had found.

"Get him in the O.R. now, I'm on my way." he replied immediately and hung up.

"Let's go! Let's go! Up to the O.R.!" I shouted to my team. Within minutes, we had the patient on the operating room table.

I had just finished shaving Antonio's head in preparation for surgery when Dr. Rashid barged in, flinging the operating room doors to the side.

"Stop! Stop! Let me examine him. Has he been given any anesthesia yet?"

"No," the anesthesiologist replied. "None yet."

I stood next to Dr. Rashid and watched as he performed his exam, similar to what I had done in the trauma bay.

While he did this, he said, "I was able to review his CT on my way in. The bleeding is significant, and the drain looks like it may have already herniated. It looks non-survivable. But he is so young … we have to try," his voice trailed off.

"Definitely," I replied, with a growing feeling of disappointment as I continued to watch him hunched over the patient.

Suddenly, Dr. Rashid stopped, stood up, and announced, "This man is not alive ... or at least his brain isn't, anyway."

The operating room was silent. Everyone had stopped what they were doing and stood as if paralyzed, letting his words sink in.

"Although his heart is still beating, has already died. He doesn't have a single brainstem reflex. His brain has died. He is no longer legally alive. I can't operate on a dead man. It won't help him. We are done here." Then, Dr. Rashid silently turned and walked out of the room, leaving us all standing there frozen, as if under a spell.

I shook myself out of what I'd hoped was a nightmare and checked the clock on the wall. "Time of death 7:12 p.m.," I announced, faintly hearing the scribbling of pens as this time was jotted down. Then I turned and followed in the direction of Dr. Rashid.

A few minutes later, Doctors Smith, Rashid, and I stood outside of the operating room.

"We need to talk to the family," Dr. Smith said. "They were at the football game. They will be here any minute." Then, to Dr. Rashid, "It would help if you were there too, to help explain why surgery wouldn't have saved him."

Dr. Rashid nodded.

Then, without thinking I repeated, "They were at the football game ...." Connecting the dots in my head I added, "That means they saw him get hit ... they saw him die ... *they watched their son die* ...." As I heard the words come out of my mouth, I felt nauseated.

Briana, one of the hospital social workers, poked her head around the corner. Seeing us, she walked over and said, "Family is here. I put them in the surgery waiting room."

"What do they know so far?" I asked.

"Nothing."

Dr. Rashid, Dr. Smith, and I followed Briana into the quiet waiting room. Inside, a man and a woman in their early forties were sitting quietly with their hands on their knees, facing us. Between them, sat two equally silent children, a boy and a girl, who looked about ten and eight.

We introduced ourselves and sat down directly across from them. As we did, all four of them watched us closely, their eyes glued to our faces, eager for any sign of good news about their son.

"Would you like to have your kids step out? I can call nurse Angie to come watch them," Briana offered.

"No, they are fine," the patient's mother replied.

Then, the patient's father cut in, "Where is Antonio? Will he have to spend the night here?"

Hearing this, I nearly fainted. These people were about to be devastated, and they had no idea.

Dr. Smith quietly cleared his throat and leaned forward, gently placing his hand on top of the patient's mother's hand. "I am sorry to have to tell you this, but your son has died."

The patient's mother raised her hands in the air and shrieked, falling forward from her chair onto her knees, holding her arms in the air, wailing, pleading with God. The father looked frantically at each one of our faces, anxiously asking if there had been some mistake, begging us to admit that there had been a mistake and that their son was still alive. The patient's mother was now lying face down on the floor, pounding it with her fists as she pleaded, her hair wet with tears and strewn around her head, her sobs now muffled by the floor. Tears had begun to fall from the corners of the father's eyes as his denial receded. Their two children sat rigid, watching this scene unfolding before them, unsure how to act. I couldn't bear what was going on. I wanted to stand up and leave but knew I couldn't. Instead, I looked down at my feet, still able to see everything through my periphery. I bit my tongue, hoping the pain wound distract me from what was going on around me. The kids started to cry, too, and soon everyone else in the room followed suit.

Rising from the floor, but still on her knees, her face ravaged from crying, the patient's mother began to grasp our hands and plead with us to save her son. Begging for us to do something more. She clutched my hands, squeezing them desperately, looking at me with her tragic eyes. It nearly broke me.

"Take me to my son," came the father's voice, shaking.

"Absolutely," came Dr. Smith's voice, and with that, Drs. Smith and Rashid led the patient's mother and father out of the room to see Antonio.

I couldn't budge. My body felt wobbly, and I wasn't sure if I would be able to stand. I looked up and noticed the two kids looking at Briana and me, the adults, expecting us to be the leaders, to tell them what to do, how to act, how to feel. I felt ashamed because I didn't know what to say or do. In that moment, I felt as lost as them.

"Was he your big brother?" came Briana's soothing voice.

The boy looked up at her and nodded.

She got up and sat next to him. "You're going to have to be her big brother now," she said, gently squeezing his hand. "You will have to be strong for the both of you now, and I am sure that you will do an amazing job."

Seven hours later, I was standing in the trauma bay again, leaning against the same counter as before, waiting. We had just been paged for another Level 1 trauma. The night had continued at a relentless pace. Time didn't stop for anything, even tragedy. My body ached from head to toe with fatigue. Throughout the entire evening, nurses had been paging me non-stop about their patients. Each time, it forced me to pull my list from my pocket, flip through it until my eyes landed on the patient in question, decipher the tiny notes I had frantically scrawled down, and then formulate an adequate response to the nurse's initial query.

"Bolus 500cc of normal saline and let me know if the urine output picks up."

"Yes, you can give them an additional dose of oxycodone."

"Why are you calling me at two a.m. to tell me they haven't had a bowel movement in the last two days? Can't this wait until morning?! You know what, never mind. Just give them a packet of Miralax."

It didn't look like I was going to get any sleep before my fellow residents showed up in two hours. Another sleepless night on call. I thought about Jeff and how he was at home sleeping, undisturbed. I yearned to be home in my bed. At that moment, I hated that I was a surgical resident. I felt like my brain was spiraling into a black hole.

"They're here, they're here!" someone shouted from the doorway.

I peeled myself up off of the counter where I had been comfortably leaning and stood up straight, trying to wake myself up. Game time.

The paramedics ran into the trauma bay pushing their gurney. Atop it was a twenty-five-year-old man wearing white Air Force One basketball shoes, blue jeans, and a black T-shirt. From head to toe, he was covered in blood. His shirt had been cut open, revealing a small hole in the front of his chest, just to the left of his breastbone. He was not moving.

As the paramedics told us what had happened, nurses worked to quickly cut off the remainder of the patient's blood-soaked clothing.

"Twenty-five-year-old man, witnesses say he was shot in the chest at least once. When we got there, he was breathing and had a pulse. His blood pressure was low on the way, so we gave him saline. We lost his pulse just now as we were wheeling him in," one of the paramedics shouted breathlessly over the sounds of scissors cutting through blue jeans.

The room had become noisy again, filled with the sounds of chaotic activity as people rushed about, preparing for what we all knew would come next.

"Check for a pulse!" Dr. Smith's voice boomed over the din.

I slapped my gloved hand down on the patient's neck and concentrated, "I don't have one!" I shouted back.

"Open the thoracotomy tray!" Dr. Smith yelled to a tech on the far side of the room. Then, leaning over my shoulder, "You want to do this one?" he asked directly into my ear.

"Yes," I replied, the rush of adrenaline coming through in my voice.

"Good."

"Give me the scalpel," I shouted to the tech who had just finished opening a sterile package titled "Thoracotomy Tray." Dr. Smith had stepped aside. I was now flying the plane.

I stuck out my hand and felt something narrow and solid being placed into it. The scalpel. I took a deep breath and then used it to cut from the patient's left breastbone toward his left arm pit, making a large curvilinear incision across the entire left side of his chest.

Since the patient did not have a pulse, he was not alive. The longer someone remains dead, the less likely it becomes that they can be revived. In these situations, every moment counts. I had to cut open his chest as fast as possible, find the source of bleeding, and stop it, all before his brain died from lack of blood flow.

I swiped the scalpel into my incision again, with each pass making it deeper. The patient's pectoralis muscles bulged out at me as I sliced through them. Just as I feared the scalpel was getting dull, I found what I had been looking for, his ribs.

"Scalpel back! Give me the rib spreader!" I shouted, handing the scalpel back to the tech, who in exchange handed me a shiny metallic set of retractors that looked like it belonged in a medieval torture chamber, not a hospital.

I jammed the sides of the retractor between two of his ribs and turned the handle as fast as I could. With each turn, the retractors spread apart, opening the tiny rib space. The room had become so loud that the associated crunch of the ribs breaking went unnoticed.

Finally, the space was large enough for me to get my hands into his chest and work. His left lung ballooned out of the incision at me, full of air, blocking my view. I pushed it out of my way, stuffing it upward in his chest to be dealt with later. I stuck my hands deep into his chest and found what I had been looking for, his heart.

With fine scissors I made an incision in the fibrous sac that contains the heart, allowing me to deliver it into my hands. To my disappointment, his heart was flat, like a deflated balloon. This was a bad sign, it meant he had already bled out. I turned his heart over in my hands and noticed a large hole on the front. I flipped it over and found a similar hole on the back. His heart had been blown to smithereens. This could not be repaired. It was amazing he had survived long enough to get to the hospital. Despite this lethal finding, we tried for twenty more minutes to resuscitate him, giving various life-saving medications, and most importantly, massive amounts of blood transfusions.

I turned and glanced over my shoulder at Dr. Smith who was still standing behind me, watching every move I made. We locked eyes and he silently shook his head. I let go of the patient's heart, glanced at the clock on the wall and said, "Time of death, 3:17 a.m." Pronouncing people dead was starting to feel all too familiar.

I pulled off my bloodied gloves and washed my hands. Blood had gotten all over my scrubs, which made me look like I had just finished butchering a cow. I needed to change. As I made my way to the locker room Dr. Smith caught up with me.

"Not bad," he said. "You need to get faster, though."

"Thank you," I replied, not sure if he was complimenting me or not.

Then, he added, "Not that it would have made much of a difference in this case, that guy was doomed. But one day, it might."

As I drove home a few hours later, I struggled to stay awake. I reflected on everything that had happened over the previous twenty-four hours: Three unlucky young men had all met their fate. The first from an unexpected and rare diagnosis of advanced-stage cancer, the second from a freak football accident, and the third at the wrong end of a gun. I mulled it over in my mind as I drove, the gentle rocking of the car threatening to put me to sleep. I finally made it home and into bed, grateful to be safe, comfortable, and at last, alone. Free from the nurses paging me, trauma activations, and grief. For now.

CHAPTER 15—I Quit

Medicine moves fast. Even though only one year had passed since Jeff had first told me of his plan to quit, it felt like years ago. Residency droned on, and even though I was approaching my fourth year, my feelings hadn't improved, not even modestly. I was stressed out and tired, and on my precious days off, all I wanted to do was sleep. I felt jealous when I'd heard how happy Jeff had become after leaving. Despite this, I still hadn't taken any serious steps toward quitting. I fantasized about quitting, but it was just a fantasy.

Meanwhile, the majority of my friends from med school had opted for three-year residencies, and while my third year would place me in the middle of my five-year residency, my friends were all preparing to graduate. My phone was constantly inundated with group text messages containing discussions speculating what life would be like after residency, when they were attending physicians. They texted about where they planned to live, how much time off they would have, and their soon-to-be salaries.

Furthermore, now that my girlfriend and I had been dating for a few years, we were becoming more serious, and I wanted to spend more time with her. It bothered me how sporadically we saw each other, and when I did, I was often exhausted and wanted to sleep. I also felt bad that I constantly cancelled plans with her at the last minute and continually missed gatherings with our friends.

"What about Saturday evening? We're all going out to celebrate Courtney's birthday. Can you come?"

"No, I'm on call that night."

"What about brunch Sunday, then?"

"I can try, but I'm going to be tired after call ... I don't want to fall asleep like last time."

"At least last time you came!"

"Sorry," I would say, annoyed that I felt like I had to apologize for being exhausted after working thirty hours straight.

"Last weekend all my friends brought their boyfriends to Carl's BBQ, I was the only one there without their boyfriend. You said you were going to come ... you owe me!"

"I told you already! I ended up having to stay late, we had to take one of our patients back to the O.R. unexpectedly." I hated feeling like I was in two full-time relationships, but I didn't want to give up either one.

"I understand."

Although she said she "understood," I knew my unreliable schedule was difficult for her. It didn't seem fair to make her suffer because of my commitment to medicine. She didn't deserve to be treated this way.

I began to realize just how many relationships around me were falling apart, and I realized that practicing medicine was a catalyst for ending relationships. One of my co-residents had already gotten divorced. Several attendings told me that they had gotten divorced during residency. To them, this was a badge of honor, awarded to them for their devotion to surgery; they were proud of the fact that they had chosen surgery over love. Other attendings were actively getting divorced, even though residency was behind them. Worse yet, the burden of medicine had prevented some from ever getting married or having a stable relationship. During surgery one afternoon I listened as the anesthesiologist and my attending surgeon Dr. Boyle chatted about this dilemma.

"They all say the same thing, that they 'get it,' but the truth is they don't," the anesthesiologist complained over the surgical drapes.

"Tell me about it," Dr. Boyle replied, standing with his arms folded across his chest while I cut, sutured, and tied. "That's why me and my wife are getting divorced."

The anesthesiologist continued, "A few months ago I met one girl who was perfect and seemed like maybe she really did 'get it.' Then, once she started staying over more, she began to get annoyed with me constantly getting paged and having to go into the hospital. Late one night I got called and had to go in, you know what she said to me?"

"What?"

"She told me to turn my pager off and just not go! Can you believe that?!"

Chuckling, "So, what happened?"

"What do you think happened? I told her that's not how it works and then we got into an argument. I left and went to work, and she went to sleep. How unfair is that?"

"Been there. Are you still seeing each other?"

"Nope. That was when I realized, she definitely did not 'get it,' so I broke up with her."

Residency was starting to wear on me, and people frequently told me to focus on the light at the end of the tunnel. Hearing conversations like these, and seeing other attending's lives fall apart through divorce and even suicide, extinguished that light.

It was the culmination of all of these things that made me finally realize why I had been feeling so miserable lately. Why I was becoming increasingly annoyed with patients, losing interest in medicine, and spending more and more time each day contemplating a career change. As the days pressed on, the web browser on my phone accumulated more and more open tabs to webpages dedicated to helping physicians leave medicine. Suddenly I realized what was going on. I was burned out. Medicine could cause me to lose not just my girlfriend, but potentially also my life. This realization added further kindling to my burning desire to quit.

Shortly thereafter, toward the end of my third year, one year after Jeff had quit, I decided I was going to follow in his footsteps. I set up a meeting with the residency program director, Dr. Moore.

Dr. Moore was a woman in her mid-fifties who had finished her surgery residency before the eighty-hour rule was widely practiced *and* during a time when surgery was still almost exclusively a boy's club. She was the last person on Earth that I wanted to admit to that surgery residency was too much for me to handle. As I walked to her office, I mentally predicted what she would say, and I resolved to not let any of her words change my mind. Enough was enough. I wanted to return to a normal life. I was done with surgery.

When I got to Dr. Moore's office, the door was already open. She was sitting behind her wooden desk looking over the tops of her glasses at a stack of papers she was holding. I knocked gently on the door.

"Come in! Come in!" she said enthusiastically without looking up. She was a high-energy person.

I stepped into the office and closed the door behind me. I started to sit down when she stuck her arm out holding the stack of papers, gesturing for me to look at them, "Take a look at this! We got another study published!" She was grinning.

"That's awesome, congratulations," came my perfunctory reply.

As I sat down, I quickly glanced around her office. There were diplomas and various other accolades hanging on the walls. On the shelf behind her were several photos of her with various people. My eyes fell on my favorite of them all, a picture of her and Barack Obama, the former president of the United States, standing together. I had always found this very impressive and somewhat intimidating. Despite her lofty personal and professional accomplishments, she was able to put anyone at ease.

"So, what can I do for you?" she asked, leaning back in her chair and looking at me. Here I was, a lowly resident, sitting in my boss's office, and she was asking me what she could do for me. Her charm was already starting to disarm me.

Before I could get my thoughts together, "I think I made a mistake" spilled out of my mouth. The irony was not lost on me. Just three years earlier I had feared it was her that had made a mistake accepting me into the residency program. Now, I was sure I had made a mistake.

"What do you mean?" she asked, leaning forward in her chair and resting her arms on her desk.

"I don't want to be a surgeon."

"Are you sure?"

"Yes."

"What do you want to be then?"

"I'm not sure." My plan was already starting to fall apart.

Dr. Moore was one of the smartest people I had ever met, cleverer than a fox. I trusted her without having to try. At that moment I found myself relying on her words to whip me back into shape. Give me a pep talk. Make me excited about surgery again. Which is why I was surprised when she said, "Well, I don't blame you. Surgery isn't for everyone. But you're still going to need to do something. So, how about this, why don't you take the weekend off and think about it. Come back to my office when you've decided what you want to do instead, and I'll do what I can to help." She came off unenthused and ambivalent, which was not what I had been expecting.

What's more, hearing these words come out of her mouth, I felt guilty. Just two years earlier, when I was a fourth-year medical student interviewing to become a resident in her program, I had sat in that same chair and told her how badly I wanted to become a surgeon. That I would do whatever it took. I would have begged if I'd had to. Now, I was sitting there again telling her the exact opposite, ready to beg to get out. She and all of the other attendings had invested time and energy into training me this far. I felt like I was letting them down.

I stood up to leave, and as if it was nothing more than an afterthought she added, "Think about what it took to get here, and what you'll be giving up. You could be a surgeon, and that's a big deal." She was no longer looking at me anymore, her attention instead returned to the papers on her desk.

I quietly left her office. The ball was in my court. She had given me the same deal she had given Jeff. All I had to do was firm up my plan a little bit and then just say the word. Developing this escape hatch took some of the pressure off. I had laid the groundwork to quit at any time I chose to. I felt like a secret agent on a mission carrying a cyanide capsule, just in case.

That night I lay in bed fantasizing about what I would do once I left surgery behind. First, I was going to get some sleep, that was a given. After that, I decided I would pursue one of my passions, photography. For the most part, gone are the days when photographers could make a living selling prints.

I would have to do something else to earn a living. Wedding photography came to mind … before I knew it, I was asleep.

CHAPTER 16—Futility

In my fourth year of residency, I became a 'senior resident.' With the change in title also came a change in my call schedule. Instead of remaining in the hospital for overnight call (in-house call), we were assigned 'home call.' This meant that at the end of each day, we could leave the hospital and go home. However, we had to remain available by phone and within twenty or so minutes of the hospital at all times. This meant that although we were allowed to go home, the activities we could participate in were limited. When on home call it was never a good idea to make dinner reservations, go for a jog ... and alcohol was absolutely out of the question.

Home call was a double-edged sword, or scalpel. In some sense it had the potential to be better than remaining in the hospital. But it was because of this that we had to do much more of it. Once I left the hospital, I was at the mercy of fate to determine how the remainder of my night would go. It was always a toss-up. On a good night, I would be disturbed only a few times by calls from the junior resident at the hospital to discuss patient care. On a bad night, I would be called back to the hospital to operate for the entire night.

The way in which the American Council on Graduate Medical Education required us to report 'home call' duty hours made accurate reporting nearly impossible. This created some interesting loopholes. For example, after home call, we were not given a 'post call day.' Normally after taking in-house call as a junior resident, once we finished our work the next morning, we were allowed to go home to sleep. This was not the case after home call, regardless of how rough the night had been. Furthermore, because of how difficult it was to track home call duty hours, combined with the fact that there were fewer senior residents (years 4 and 5) than junior residents (years 1, 2, and 3), we had to take home call more frequently than we'd had to take in-house call as junior residents. If senior residents were on away rotations or on vacation, the remaining senior residents had to take even more frequent calls to fill the gap. This is how I got stuck covering an entire weekend of home call by myself.

It was Friday, the end of a long week. I was exhausted, and after getting home I went straight to bed and immediately fell asleep. That was one of the nice things about residency and being constantly tired. While the rest of America lay in bed at night staring at their cellphones wishing they could fall asleep, I never once had any difficulties getting to sleep. Whenever friends or family members asked me what to do about their difficulties sleeping, I always (half) jokingly told them that I was going to prescribe them more 'call.' Throughout residency, uninterrupted sleep became the most valuable commodity that any of us could possess. It was coveted by all. We would go to great lengths to oppose last minute schedule changes that impinged on our ability to get a full night's worth of rest, at times alienating each other in an attempt to protect our precious privilege to sleep. We craved for shut eye like a mouse craves cheese.

That night, immediately after I had dozed off, my junior resident Gabriella called me and told me that a patient at the hospital needed surgery right away. As I always did when I was pulled from sleep by an emergency at the hospital, I sat in bed for about five minutes debating in my mind going to the hospital or going back to sleep instead. Then finally, I threw off the covers, walked across my bedroom in the dark, and pulled on my scrubs that I had left hanging on my bedroom door for me to easily find in exactly this scenario.

After we finished surgery, around one a.m., I snuck downstairs to the in-house resident call room. I decided that I would be able to get more sleep if I stayed at the hospital instead of driving back home, since I would have to be back at the hospital early that morning to round anyway. I crept into one of the abandoned call rooms and lay on top of the stiff bed and rested my head against the flat plastic pillow. I had just closed my eyes when my phone rang.

As if sensing what I was doing and not wanting to allow it to happen, Gabriella called me and told me that there was another patient that needed surgery, a trauma patient this time. I had really been hoping to get some sleep, but this was not going to be that kind of night. And it was only the first of three in a row.

"What happened?" I said into the phone, frustrated, hoping that I could come up with some sort of reasonable non-operative plan instead that would allow me to get some sleep instead of operating.

"Shot in the abdomen. Hypotensive. Positive FAST exam. Needs to go now," she related back to me matter-of-factly.

"Great," I replied, making no attempt to hide my sarcasm. There was definitely no way to justify not operating on this person.

I propped my head up against the wall and blinked my eyes a few times. Gabriella didn't know that I was still in the hospital. She probably though that I had gone back home. This would allow me time to at least complete my five-minute routine of lying there, debating getting up or going back to sleep. It's a pointless exercise since I always end up going. But in this case, the routine served another, darker, purpose as well. From Gabriella's description of the patient, I knew they were in very bad shape. So bad in fact, that it was likely they would die any minute. If this happened, then I could go back to sleep.

I know what you are thinking, how horrible of a thought this was for me to have. And I agree with you, it was. But I include it here to emphasize how important sleep, something most people take for granted, becomes to a person once it is has been taken away. It changes people. I also want to assure you, that by remaining in bed, I did NOT contribute to this patient's demise in any way by delaying care. I knew that Gabriella was at the patient's bedside with one of the attending trauma surgeons and did not need my help at that moment getting the patient up to the operating room.

Twice so far that night I had been awaken just after falling asleep. Each time this happened it hurt more, causing physical pain to my entire body.

140

As had become custom for me, I thought jealously about how the rest of the world was fast asleep in bed. This, of course, only upset me.

When I got upstairs to the O.R. I paused at the front desk and noticed a blood-soaked gurney just outside of O.R. 2, the dedicated trauma room at night. The white sheets had been stained red and blood was dripping off of the gurney onto the floor making a splattering sound. Through the tiny vertical windows on the double doors of O.R. 2, I indistinctly saw figures busily scurrying about preparing the patient for surgery, their commotion muffled by the doors. To most, the scene would look like one straight out of a horror film, but in trauma surgery, it was typical.

Despite the fact that I had been *here* before many times by the time I was a senior resident, I needed an additional minute to mentally prepare for what lay behind those doors. Furthermore, I needed to calm down. I was frustrated that I wouldn't be getting another opportunity to sleep that night. I needed a second to convince my mind that, like I had many times before, I would survive. I wanted to walk into the room as collected and composed as possible. Rushing into a situation like this worked up, excited, shaking, with your mind elsewhere, is a recipe for disaster. In surgery, it is important not to rush. Through experience, I have found that rushing will always do the opposite of what is intended. Like a drowning person flailing their arms and legs, rushing inevitably leads to mistakes and mistakes lead to slow downs. Instead, to be fast, one must operate quickly, methodically, thoughtfully, each move deliberate, never rushed. This is a lesson that since learning I have successfully applied to other facets of my life.

I leaned against the O.R. desk and put on boot covers. Boot covers are like shoe covers except that they come up nearly to your knee, providing extra protection. They take a little bit more effort to put on than shoe covers, but whenever I don't wear them, and I feel my socks get soggy with patient's blood during surgery, I always wish I had taken the extra minute. This was another lesson that wasn't in any textbook and only comes with experience.

Finally, I stepped into the operating room, plunging headfirst into the chaos. There was no turning back now. I was finally mentally prepared and physically present. I took stock of everything that was going on. Gabriella and Dr. Ferguson, the attending trauma surgeon on call that night, had just finishing placing the surgical drapes over the patient. The anesthesiologist was moving rapidly about at the head of the bed, two red picnic coolers with their lids open at his feet. These coolers are called *MTP* coolers, or *Massive Transfusion Protocol* coolers, and are identical to the one you might take with you on a picnic, except that these are filled with bags of blood instead of beer and sandwiches.

From these coolers, nurses were hurriedly pulling out bags of red blood and yellow plasma, confirming the blood type, which was printed in large letters on each bag, and then feeding them into the *rapid transfuser*. The *rapid transfuser* is a machine used to rapidly warm and squeeze an entire unit of blood into a patient in less than thirty seconds. Once its contents had been transfused, the nurse running the machine would take the empty bag of blood out and throw it onto a growing pile of empty blood bags on the ground. Later these bags would be counted so that we'd know how many units of blood the patient had required. I glanced at the rapidly growing pile of empty blood bags on the floor. This was the real deal.

I quickly washed my hands, bypassing the scrub tank, using Avagard instead, a shiny white chemical that is designed to replace the time-consuming process of scrubbing and rapidly sterilize surgeon's hands prior to surgery. After donning my surgical attire, I stepped up to the table on the patient's left across from Dr. Ferguson, pushing the curious Gabriella and medical student out of my way toward the patient's feet. This operation would require experienced hands.

They had just finished opening the abdomen and blood was pouring out over the sides of the bed. I was glad that I had taken the extra time to put on the boot covers. As fast as we could, we systematically shoved surgical sponges into every part of the patient's abdomen, a technique designed to compress the source of bleeding, wherever it may be, temporarily stopping it.

Once we had the abdomen fully packed, we paused. All of the blood that was being transfused into the patient had been exiting through whatever was bleeding in the patient's abdomen. Definitely something large. With the bleeding temporarily under control, now was a good time to allow the rest of the team to *catch up* and transfuse more blood.

This was the eye of the storm. Our packing created a temporary break for Dr. Ferguson and me to devise a plan. Up until then we had not spoken yet. We both knew the first parts of the operation well and didn't need to discuss each step. Dr. Ferguson, who had first seen the patient when he first arrived, told me that he had been shot in both the groin and the lower right part of his abdomen. Confirming what I already knew, she told me that he had been in bad shape when he arrived, and that she was concerned about a major vascular injury. Based on the amount of blood that has poured out of his abdomen, so was I.

While the team caught up, we quickly examined the portions of the abdomen that remained exposed through our surgical sponges and discovered a large hole in the colon, spewing stool into the surgical field where it mixed with the patient's blood, creating a thick foul-smelling soup. I grabbed a bowel stapler and quickly removed the segment of damaged bowel.

After a few minutes and several more units of blood had been transfused, we started removing the surgical sponges we had placed inside the abdomen. We turned our attention specifically to the right lower quadrant where the patient had been shot, and where we suspected the offending injury to be. The moment we removed our packing from it, the patient's entire pelvis and abdomen filled with dark blood.

The problem with blood is that unlike other liquids like water, it is not transparent. When it accumulates, it hides beneath it the source of bleeding. Without being able to see where exactly the bleeding is coming from, it becomes impossible to surgically address the problem. Meanwhile, the bleeding continues. A deadly loop that must be broken. It becomes a race between our *rapid transfuser* and the hole in the patient's blood vessel.

Dr. Ferguson stuck her hand into the pool of blood and pushed down, hoping to be able to blindly compress and slow the bleeding vessel. By now, it was clear that it was probably the iliac artery or vein (or maybe both) that were damaged, two blood vessels that are notoriously difficult to get to and fix.

As she felt around with her fingers trying to slow the bleeding, I stuck two suction devices into the pool of blood attempting to clear away as much as possible, potentially giving us a glimpse of the damaged vessel below. As long as the suction devices were removing the blood faster than it was accumulating, this would work.

Initially nothing happened, but as Dr. Ferguson continued to move her hand around, submerged in the pool of blood, the blood finally started to clear. This meant that her hand had found the area of the injury and was effectively controlling the bleeding, or at least slowing it. A temporary fix.

In order to fix the hole however, she would eventually need to move her hand. But each time she moved her hand in the slightest, the blood would rapidly re-accumulate, and we would be back at square one. We couldn't find a good opportunity to throw a stitch. Compounding the problem further is the fact that the pelvis is a tight space, the bowl-like pelvic bone restricts the room there is for us to introduce additional hands or instruments to help.

Every time she removed her hand and one of us tried to throw a stitch, the patient would immediately lose about three units of blood and we would have to start all over. We were limited in the number of times we could try this because three units per second was faster than we could transfuse him, even with our rapid transfuser. And each time he lost more blood than we could replace, his blood pressure would get lower and lower, ultimately bringing him closer and closer to death. What we were doing wasn't working. Continuing in this way would be insanity.

After our third try, we stopped and held pressure. It was clear what we were doing wasn't going to work. We needed to come up with a better plan. We needed to get better control of the vessel that was bleeding and occlude it in front of the hole that was bleeding. Like kinking a hose. This would allow us to visualize the hole without blood pouring out of it and fix it. But like I mentioned before, the iliac artery and vein are two notoriously difficult vessels to expose, and control buried deep within the confines of the tight pelvis space.

We began working in the patient's abdomen, identifying first his aorta, the major blood vessel that carries blood away from the heart. From the aorta all other blood vessels arise, and we were going to attempt to trace the origin of the iliac artery from it.

Once we found it, we placed an elastic vessel loop, like a rubber band, around it. Just behind the iliac artery is the iliac vein and we placed a vessel loop around this too. This temporary slowed the bleeding, simultaneously stopping all blood flow going into the patient's pelvis and right leg beyond. In the back of our minds, we knew this was another temporary measure, we could only occlude this vessel cutting off circulation to his leg for so long before it died.

The vessel loops we had placed near the origin of the vessels has succeeded in slowing the bleeding but not stopping it completely. The hole was still bleeding too briskly to repair due to back bleeding from the leg. This meant that we would also have to dissect the vessel beyond the hole and occlude it there as well. This entire process is called *getting proximal and distal control*.

To do this, I made a large vertical incision up the front of the patient's right leg, crossing the crease in his groin. I quickly and carefully dissected through the fatty tissue underneath the skin until I found the femoral vessels, the leg vessels that the iliac artery and vein became. I placed similar elastic vessel loops around them, theoretically occluding all blood flow from crossing the site of injury in the pelvis and creating a blood free environment for us to repair the injury. If our estimations were correct, then Dr. Ferguson should be able to remove her hand from the injury and there would be no further bleeding, bestowing on us a clear view, like the clouds clearing after a storm revealing a tranquil ocean.

In reality, though, we knew this would not be the case. There are always small unnamed vessels called collaterals that connect to all of the larger vessels allowing *some* blood to still pass through. Our hope was not that the bleeding would be completely stopped, but that it would be slowed enough to allow us long enough glimpses of the hole to get a stitch in it.

She removed her hand, and as hoped, we got our first look at the injury. We were not pleased with what we saw. Our worst suspicions were confirmed. Both the iliac artery and vein had been damaged. But there wasn't a discrete hole like we had been hoping. Instead, the entire sides of both vessels had been torn off by the bullet. This tear extended from inside the patient's pelvis all the way down into his leg. This type of injury is much more complex to fix than a simple hole.

We needed a new plan, and fast. The longer we spent in the operating room, the more dire the patient's situation would become. Already he was beginning to show signs of a life-threatening condition called D.I.C.

D.I.C. is short for *Disseminated Intravascular Coagulopathy,* or more sinisterly, *Death Is Coming.* In short, what this means is that the patient has lost their ability to properly form blood clots. When this happens, patients begin to bleed from all over, even places they weren't bleeding from initially—IV sites, their gums, lungs, nose, etc.— and especially from the site of injury. D.I.C. is a poorly understood phenomena that can happen to patients with deadly infections, pregnancy, and especially trauma patients who have required massive amounts of transfusion. Worst of all, due to the diffuse nature of this type of bleeding, it is impossible to stop with surgery. That is why, when operating on severely injured trauma patients, it is imperative to move as fast as possible. A trauma operation is a race against time to get out of the O.R. before D.I.C. sets in. The longer a trauma surgeon spends operating, the more likely it becomes that D.I.C. will develop and kill their patient. This is what was happening to our patient now in front of our eyes.

Reading our thoughts, the anesthesiologist shouted from underneath the drapes at the head of the patient's bed, "I've got a lot of blood starting to come out of his endotracheal tube. I think he's going into D.I.C.!"

We needed to get out of the O.R. immediately, our patient's life depended on it. We converted to a damage control operation and accepted the fact that we could not fix his damaged blood vessels at this time. We transected the veins that we had placed vessel loops around (veins can almost always be transected without major impact later one) and put *shunts,* small straws meant to temporarily connect one end of an artery to the other, into his damaged artery. For the time being, this would allow enough blood flow to his leg to prevent it from dying.

Because he was in D.I.C., he continued to ooze a substantial amount in his pelvis from the raw surfaces of his wound. To combat this, we re-packed new surgical sponges into his pelvis against all of the raw wound edges, stopping the bleeding for the time being. We forwent formally sewing closed the large abdominal wound we had created, instead covering it with a specially designed clear sheet of plastic, which could be done more quickly. In this way we performed an abbreviated operation. None of these measures were intended to be a permanent. Only *if*, after being taken to the ICU, the patient recovered from D.I.C. and survived, would we return to the operating room and attempt finish what we had started. By now it was around three a.m. I helped the nurses move the patient to the ICU.

In the ICU, several police officers were milling around. Upon seeing me, one of them immediately came over and asked if I thought the patient would survive or not. This information helps them decide whether their crime scene is a homicide or not.

I told the officer that the patient was "alive but in critical condition," and he could very well take a turn for the worse at any moment. The officer thanked me and then spoke into his radio, "Call the detectives, sounds like you boys are going to need to prepare for a homicide investigation."

As I typically do, I chatted with the officers for a bit, attempting to find out what had happened to our patient leading to him getting shot. The officers told me that there had been a shooting at a bar nearby. My mind jumped straight to the bar on the corner of the five-way intersection which contributed endlessly to drumming up business for our trauma center in one way or another.

Then, in a more hushed tone, he added that the lobby of our hospital was beginning to fill up with the patient's "friends and family," making air quotes with his fingers. He continued, saying that nearly all of them were known to be affiliated with a local biker gang. The police advised us to limit the number of visitors allowed to come see the patient for fear that further violence could occur, especially if rival gang members came and tried to finish the job.

With this information, we agreed to let only two people come visit initially: the patient's mother and sister. Security guards were sent downstairs to fetch them and bring them upstairs to the patient's room in the ICU. When they arrived, they were sobbing hysterically. His sister's pants were covered in blood which made me wonder if she was with her brother when he had been shot. I was sure the detectives would have some questions for her later.

Despite our attempted imposition on visitors, about six more people somehow found their way past security and upstairs to the ICU. They all stood back from the patient's bed as if scared to approach, and then took turns going to his bedside and saying things to him. I was not able to hear what they were saying. Perhaps they were reassuring the patient that everything would be ok or promising him that they would seek revenge.

While this was going on, I had been closely monitoring the patient's vital signs and I started to notice that the patient was getting worse instead of better. He was still needing a large amount of blood transfusions and was on his sixth picnic cooler-full of bags of blood. The clear plastic that we had placed over his open abdomen had begun to swell as it strained to contain blood welling up beneath it.

By five a.m., we knew we had to take him back to the operating room. Our temporary attempts at controlling the bleeding were clearly no longer working, and despite the D.I.C., we would have to try again. This time, once we got into the O.R., we called in another trauma surgeon to see if they had any ideas that we might have overlooked. On the phone, we explained the situation to him. He didn't have any great advice for us and wished us luck.

We threw a few blind stitches into the patient's pelvis and replaced the packing again with similar results as the first time. Only this time, instead of taking the patient to the ICU, we planned to take him to I.R., the Interventional Radiology suite. Here, a radiologist would inject dye into his vessels and, using X-rays, follow the dye to see where the vessel was bleeding so that another chemical could be injected to occlude the vessel from the inside preventing more bleeding. It was a last-ditch plan.

I stepped out of the room and stood in the O.R. hallway to catch my breath while the nurses got the patient off of the O.R. table and prepared to move him downstairs. As I stood there, one of the hospital's spine surgeons, Dr. Clearwater—an older man shorter than me, with long frizzy hair—came up and stood next to me. He followed my gaze through the rectangular windows in the O.R. doors and together we watched the nurses move the patient off of the blood-soaked operating room onto a clean gurney. I wondered why he was here in the middle of the night. Then, I realized that it was morning; we had been working all night. He was probably there to begin his seven-thirty a.m. elective surgeries. Realizing this, I felt tired again and my entire body began to ache.

Dr. Clearwater, gazing curiously into the operating room, asked me what had happened to the patient. I quickly recounted what the police had told me, that there had been a gang shooting. Then I told him about the iliac artery and vein injury, to which he sighed and said, "Bad luck, those are tough."

I brought him up to speed, finishing off by telling him how we had been transfusing him all night while we had tried to get the bleeding to stop and that we were now going to try going to I.R.

He told me that when he had shown up for work that morning the hospital lobby had been packed with bikers. I told him that I had heard that as well. Then he added, "The blood bank doesn't have infinite blood, you know?"

"I know."

"What do you do if another trauma patient comes in right now and needs a blood transfusion and the blood bank is out because you used it all on this guy? What about them?", he added, almost accusatory.

He went on, "Who pays for all of this anyways?"

Again, I didn't say anything.

He kept going; he was on a roll now—ranting is a favorite surgical past time— "A gang shooting right? What about the average guy driving to work this morning who gets hit by a drunk driver coming home from that same bar and he needs a transfusion but can't get one because there is no more blood left, because you used it all up trying to save this gang banger who wanted to get drunk and have a gun fight instead of going to sleep like the rest of us?"

He paused to let his reverberation sink in, then continued, "At what point does it become futile?"

I shrugged and didn't say anything. He slapped me on the back, smiling now that he had finished extolling onto me his thoughts. "Tough question, huh?" Before I had the chance to agree, he walked away wishing me "good luck" over his shoulder. I didn't care about a single thing he had just said. All I could think about at that moment was how jealous I was that while I had been up all night, he had been asleep and was just now beginning his day.

Downstairs in the interventional radiology suite, the patient continued to do horribly. He continued to bleed, and his heart stopped a few times, and each time we had to perform CPR, breaking his ribs, and shock him to get it started again. As I sat behind the lead re-enforced glass watching the interventional radiologist work, I began to hallucinate.

This happens to me when I have been awake for long periods of time. Things I looked at would change shapes, and if I kept looking, they would continue to do so until one of two things happened: 1) The changes would become so bizarre that I would realize I was starting to dream while I was still awake and could snap myself out of it, or 2) I would start to nod off completely, falling over, only to be woken up by the sensation of falling. Both of these happened multiple times while I waited behind the glass in the interventional radiology suite.

Just like us in the O.R., the I.R. doctor was unable to find the source of bleeding. Like us, there was nothing the I.R. doctor could fix. This was because the patient was now in florid D.I.C., bleeding from everywhere. He was alive, but he was doomed. Death was coming.

We took him back to the ICU and transfused him in the hopes that he would turn a corner. The family was there and was crying and begging for everything to be done to keep him alive, which we were doing.

It was around this time, one of the general surgeons—Dr. Gerard—called me. He was looking for the on-call resident to help him take out part of a patient's colon that had perforated. I told him that I was the resident on call, mentioning none of the night's events.

I joined him in the O.R. As I donned my surgical gown and gloves, I heard a code blue called overhead. Someone's heart somewhere in the hospital had stopped beating. About thirty minutes later, while Dr. Gerard and I were absorbed in the current operation, the intern from the ICU came into the room and told me that my patient had just died.

"Thanks," I said, dismissing him without taking any of my focus off of our current operation.

We finished the operation around four p.m. Toward the end of the surgery, I started to rush and made a mistake that cost us thirty extra minutes of work. It was a careless mistake, and I felt bad. I was annoyed with myself; I knew better than to rush.

I was exhausted and my mood soured further as I thought about how I was still on call again that night, *and* the next day, *and* the next night and so on and so forth until the weekend was over, and the other senior residents returned from wherever they had gone. As I thought about it, I began to panic a little bit that I might not get to sleep again for several days. Despite that fact that I had always been able to survive call before, I started to worry that this time I might not be able to.

And for what? The patient I had been operating on all night, spending all of the hospital's resources on, had just died.

In the surgery recovery room Dr. Gerard came and found me where I was sitting writing the post-operative orders for the patient we had just finished operating on. He told me he was on call with me that night and told me to go home. There was still another patient left that needed surgery, but he said it was minor, and he would do it alone. The classic surgical response would be to argue with him that I wanted to stay, saying things like "I'll sleep when I die." But we both knew how tired I was. It was obvious looking at me.

I went home and showered, savoring the sensation of the layers of sweat and grease accumulated over the long night, wash off of my body, making me feel clean again. There was blood coating my legs that had apparently soaked through my scrubs that I hadn't noticed before. Then I collapsed into my bed. I didn't set an alarm. If anyone needed me, they would call me, and I would answer. If I had to go back to the hospital, I would sit up in bed for five minutes and my mind would do the dance it has done so many times before, knowing that in the end, I would go.

CHAPTER 17—Every Day is a Gift

I t was a bright Tuesday morning in the spring of my fourth year. As I walked from the parking lot into the hospital, I noticed the beautiful flowers that the indigenous cacti produce. Seemingly overnight the various cacti had exploded with various colorful flowers, creating a nice disruption to the usual earthy desert beiges and browns. I'd never noticed this before in my four years in Phoenix. I stopped to examine one, a large white flower that extended outward from the top of a three-foot Saguaro, like a trumpet. I smiled. Although the ups and downs of residency still plagued me, I felt more at ease knowing that I had a way out. I was able to stop focusing on how many days were left in residency, and I began to wonder what my life would be like afterward. For now, I was able to focus on living day to day.

For the previous two weeks I had been rotating at another hospital across town, doing a rotation in a niche surgical subspecialty related to liver and pancreatic cancer, known as hepatopancreaticobiliary surgery. It had been nice to be away from my home hospital for a little while.

Mid-morning, I was sitting in the small office that I shared with five other residents adjacent to the surgery clinic's patient exam rooms. I was staring at the images from a CT scan done for the patient I was about to see. I was perplexed. I could clearly see a large mass extending upward from the patient's pancreas, wrapping itself around the stomach, squeezing, constricting it, making it nearly impossible for food to pass through. This was the worst case of pancreatic cancer I had ever seen. Clearly unresectable, meaning that surgery wouldn't help.

Why was this patient here? I wondered. *The referring physician should have known there was nothing that we could do to help.*

As I continued to scroll through the images, I wondered if there was anything at all we could do to help the patient. Dr. Nik, head of the department, appeared in my office doorway. He was a large man whose presence was immediately noticeable. He had forearms the size of bowling pins, a shiny bald head to match, and a thick Russian accent. If it wasn't for his long white lab coat, which extended well past his knees, he could have easily been mistaken for a Russian mobster. Despite his imposing figure, his demeanor was as gentle as a kitten.

"Why is she here?" he asked in his thick accent, looking over my shoulder at the CT scan on my computer screen. "Clearly unresectable."

"I don't know," I replied.

"Let's go see her and figure this out. I've got a meeting in fifteen minutes, so let's be quick."

We walked down the clinic hallway to the exam room where the patient was waiting. Dr. Nik knocked on her door, and without waiting for a reply he opened it, and we both stepped in. There were already three people in the fluorescent-lit room.

Sitting upright on the thin paper that covered the examination table was the patient, a forty-one-year-old underweight woman with dark brown hair. She was dressed casually, wearing jeans and a flowery button up shirt. Both her jeans and shirt looked to be too big for her, the result of sudden weight loss. From reviewing her medical records, I knew that she had never had a medical problem before in her life. She had been a stranger to doctor's offices until about six months ago, when she abruptly started losing weight. Now, she was a regular. Amazingly, she was smiling.

Sitting across the linoleum floor from the patient was her husband and her sister. Her husband was sitting upright in his chair with his arms folded across his chest. He was wearing a polo shirt, khaki shorts, and a poker face. The patient's sister, however, wore the expression of a someone who was grief-stricken. She looked as if she was on the verge of tears.

Dr. Nik sat down on the adjacent round stool that doctors always sit on, the bottom of his long white coat grazing the floor. The room was quiet. I stood in the corner, a fly on the wall, waiting for the silence to break.

Now that he was eye level with everyone in the room, Dr. Nik looked directly into the patient's eyes, and in a soft voice filled with genuine interest, he said, "Tell me what happened ..."

No longer able to hold it in, the patient's sister immediately burst into tears. Dr. Nik produced a tissue seemingly from nowhere, and sat patiently, as if he had all the time in the world.

"We know it's bad," the patient cut in. "The doctors at our hospital told us that surgery was the only option left, the only shot at a cure ..." her voice trailed off.

Respectfully, as if he was speaking to his own mother, Dr. Nik asked, "Why didn't *they* do surgery?"—referring to the hospital that had told the patient she needed surgery but refused to do it.

"They told us it was unresectable."

"I see," Dr. Nik said thoughtfully, as if considering this for the first time.

Slowly, he leaned over, placed both of his elbows on his knees and pressed the palms of his hands together as if he was going to pray, and then he rested his chin on his fingertips pensively. Doing this made his face level with the patient, and they locked eyes. Knowingly, as if he was a detective who had already solved the crime, he guided the conversation, "And then what? Did *they* send you here?"

There was a pause. The air in the room was still and the lights felt like they had gotten brighter. The patient's sister sobbed quietly as she continued, "Well, not quite. I was at home watching TV one day when an advertisement came on for your clinic. They showed a man who said that he had pancreatic cancer that was unresectable. He said he went to your clinic, and they resected it, and now he's cured! After I saw that, I called my sister right away and we got on a plane and came here."

Although this clinic visit was a big deal for the patient and her family, I knew that Dr. Nik had encounters like this all the time. I was amazed at how skillfully he hid this fact, respectfully listening to the patient and her family

154

tell a story I was sure he had heard before. He could easily have walked in the room and said "I reviewed the CT scan. There's nothing I can do to help you. Have a great day," and left, making it to his meeting on time. But he didn't do that.

"I see," Dr. Nik said patiently leaning back on his stool, resting his back against the wall. He folded his arm across his chest, the fingers of his left hand massaged his chin thoughtfully.

There was another pause. The patient's husband spoke for the first time, "Please, help us."

Dr. Nik didn't say anything right away, but I knew what he was thinking. In his head, he was upset that in order to survive, the hospital had to function like a business, occasionally having to advertise its product: hope. In this case however, there would be no "sale." The advertisement had misled this family and had unintentionally given them false hope. Sitting here, face to face with this dying woman and her distraught family, it was now Dr. Nik's job to tell them that. The hospital administrators who had commissioned the advertisement would not come and explain the misunderstanding. There was only him. He had to be the one to look each one of them in the eyes and tell them that despite whatever they had seen or heard, there was nothing more that could be done. This burden fell entirely on him.

He sat quietly, considering. Then he unfolded his arms, nodded slowly, and said, "Let's look at her CT scan together."

Over the next thirty minutes we all gathered around Dr. Nik as he scrolled through the CT scan images, explaining each one as he did. The edges of his white coat danced on the linoleum floor as moved his arms, pointing to things on the screen. He carefully explained why the tumor was unresectable and why she would be worse off with an operation than without one. He apologized that they had come all this way, and that he couldn't help them. He told them he really wished he could.

The patient and her family cried, passed around the tissues, and everyone blew their noses. Finally, Dr. Nik stood up, and as he did, so did everyone else in the room. They hugged and thanked him. He hadn't cured her cancer, but he had done something that no one else had. He had taken the time to help them understand, and by doing so, he had given them the closure that everyone else had been too afraid to. And for that, they were grateful.

He told them to take as long as they needed, and then he stepped out of the room, and I followed him back down the clinic hallway. Halfway down the hall, just to break the silence I said, "You're late for your meeting."

The second the words had left my mouth he stopped, turned, and faced me. He locked his eyes with mine. The intensity of his stare pushed me back against the wall and held me there, frozen. Out of my peripheral vision I could see his hands at the ends of his large forearms were clenched into fists, but I knew he wasn't mad at me. Then, very slowly, he said; "Every day is a gift. Don't ever forget that."

With that, he turned and continued on, disappearing around a corner.

Although I was unaware of it at the time, I was about to serendipitously gain two mentors who would change my outlook entirely and save me from quitting.

Because of Dr. Diaz's comment on our first day of residency— "Attendings are not here to be your friend."—I typically walked on eggshells around attending surgeons, people who I would spend countless hours with. I ensured that all of my interactions with them were strictly professional. Rarely did I make any inquiries into their personal lives. I was careful never to ask prodding questions like, "How was your weekend?" I did not want to violate the terms of our relationship, which had been so clearly defined on day one. I didn't want anyone to mistakenly think that I was trying to become their friend. It was a cold relationship. They were my bosses, and I was there to work and learn. But rules are meant to be broken.

When I was teetering on the edge of quitting residency, the hospital hired a new attending surgeon, Dr. Chowhurdy. Dr. Chowhurdy had just finished his surgery residency and was only a few years older than me. On his first day, I had been assigned to show him around the hospital. I spent the morning with him making small talk and showing him where all the important things were: the operating room, secret bathrooms, ending the tour at the most important landmark of all, the cafeteria, where we stopped and had lunch.

Dr. Chowhurdy was gregarious and engaging.

"You decide what type of surgeon you want to be yet?" he asked me over lasagna.

This is a common question throughout residency. It ranks up there with "Where are you from?" I felt guilty that I was considering quitting, and I didn't want to let him down so soon after meeting, so I replied with the most noncommittal response I could think of: "A good one."

He chuckled, "Duh," but he wasn't going to let me off the hook that easily. "Any particular specialty?"

I thought about it for a moment then said, "Trauma."

"Yeah, I heard you guys do a lot of trauma here."

"We do. I feel like I would be good at it."

"That's cool. What do you like to do for fun?" I remembered Dr. Diaz's lecture on the first day of residency: The attendings are not our friends.

Was this a trap? Was he trying to be friends with me? Had he not gotten *the lecture* yet?

Trap or not, I took the bait. "I'm really into photography."

"Awesome, dude. Any particular type?"

"Astrophotography. It's like landscape photography, but at night, so it includes the stars and the Milky Way."

"No way! Show me some!"

I pulled out my phone and scrolled through some recent photos I had taken. "Arizona is great for this sort of thing because once you get out into the desert, there's hardly any light pollution."

The rest of lunch went on like that, both of us opening up about ourselves. He told me how he had moved to the US, what residency on the East Coast had been like, and even about a recent failed relationship he had just gotten out of. I was stunned at the way he talked to me like an equal.

We immediately became friends. Moreover, Dr. Chowhurdy had a strong passion for surgery, and was very good at it too. His combination of likability and surgical skill inspired me, and that helped to broaden my narrowed perspective of surgery. I felt my attitude toward the profession start to brighten. If he could survive residency and still be cool, then so could I.

My second mentor was even more unlikely. Dr. Stillmann was a white-haired surgeon in his early sixties who had completed his surgical training decades ago, in an era when the term "well-being" didn't even exist yet. Because of this, I had been certain he shared Dr. Diaz's views on the attending-resident relationship. I was terrified of him. He had a matter-of-fact manner that came off as harsh and unfriendly. Furthermore, he had a reputation for yelling in the O.R. and kicking residents out if they couldn't correctly identify anatomical structures during the operation. Every time I set foot into the O.R. with him I feared I was going to relive my first failed anatomy practical all over again. As a result, I kept my head down around him and was especially careful never to make any inquiries into his private life. I became an expert at tiptoeing.

As I continued to advance through residency, I operated with him frequently. As we spent more time together operating, we also ended up spending more time together between cases. Despite my best efforts to minimize small talk, to my sheer terror, one day we ended up discussing our hobbies.

We were sitting in the surgeon's lounge (a small room near to the operating rooms with couches, a TV, coffee maker, and refrigerator where surgeons hang out in between cases if they aren't seeing consults) late one morning waiting for the O.R. to be turned over and set up for our next case. We were sitting quietly, only half paying attention to the TV, as it blared the news.

"Check this out," Dr. Stillmann said to me, pulling a bag out from behind one of the couches.

I leaned forward curiously and watched as he unzipped the top of the bag and extracted something large.

"I took these a month ago when I was in Antarctica," he said, handing me a stack of 24x30-inch black and white photographs printed on glossy paper. "I just got my printer working again. Tell me what you think."

You were in Antarctica?! I thought, stunned. I slowly leafed through the stack of photographs, carefully examining each one. There were beautiful pictures of icebergs floating listlessly in the cold ocean, whales showing off their tails, and penguins waddling around.

"You shoot?" I asked, as I looked through the photos, knowing the answer was obviously yes.

"Yup," he said watching me.

"I really like this one," I said, turning the photograph toward him so that he could see which one I was looking at. "I like the way this iceberg looks like it is gesturing. It really brings it to life."

"Thank you, that's one of my favorite ones as well."

"What camera do you use?"

"Nikon D850."

"No way, I've been considering upgrading to that camera!" I said excitedly, beginning to forget the rules about being friendly with attendings.

"It's a great camera, I really like mine. If you want, I can bring it in later this week so you can check it out."

"That would be awesome!"

A nurse stuck her head the doorway of the lounge. "Stillmann! They're waiting for you in O.R. 5, patient's asleep!" she said loudly before walking away. Her interruption brought me crashing back to Earth.

I handed the photographs back to Dr. Stillmann and hurried over to O.R. 5 while he replaced them in his bag. I needed to make sure the drapes were placed correctly on the sleeping patient before Dr. Stillmann arrived.

Aside from the toll that residency was taking on my life, one of the main reasons that I had wanted to quit was because I had the impression that a career in surgery was all-consuming and left no time for hobbies. That is why it was so shocking to me to learn that Dr. Stillman not only had hobbies, but *cool* ones. Aside from riding motorcycles and whitewater rafting, Dr. Stillman, like me, was also an avid photographer. He traveled to all ends of the planet taking pictures, from Iceland to Antarctica. From then on, we spent countless hours between surgeries and over lunch discussing new cameras, secret photography locations, editing, and of course, sharing our pictures with each other.

Contrary to what Dr. Diaz had probably feared would happen, being friends with Dr. Stillman never compromised the quality of my training. If anything, it improved it. I looked up to Dr. Stillman even more than I did before when I had thought he was *only* a surgeon. As a result, I worked harder and strived not to disappoint him. To this day, I still utilize a number of valuable surgical techniques that he taught me when we operated together.

Drs. Chowhurdy and Stillman had something else in common. While most surgeons discouraged residents from having hobbies, wanting them instead to focus all of their time and energy on learning surgery, they did the opposite, they *encouraged* it. As scandalous as this recommendation was, they were right. In the end, having outlets through which to mentally escape the horrors of the hospital turned out to be essential for me to maintain my sanity and recharge my resolve and desire to finish residency.

CHAPTER 18—The Enemy of Good

Very often in our lives we see things that we think we understand, but it is not until much later that we realize otherwise. And when we do, it can cause us to question everything else we thought we knew for sure. This happened to me when I was a third-year medical student, and it took nearly five years for me to realize.

"There's an ectopic pregnancy in the E.D. right now!" I blurted out excitedly to the attending OB-GYN on call.

He looked at me, clearly annoyed. "Do you honestly think that there is a single thing in this hospital right now that you know about that I don't?" he immediately retorted back to me, through a German accent.

There is no nice way to say it, but Dr. Jaggers is a dick, especially to medical students, or anyone else he deems as an annoyance. But he was who was on call and who I was assigned to work with. It would have suited him just fine if I had holed myself up out of site and studied quietly until it was time for me to go home, like most of the other med students did when they rotated with him. But that wasn't what I wanted. I was gung-ho to become a surgeon and eager to get into the operating room as much as possible. Ectopic pregnancies needed surgery, and my texts books would still be waiting for me afterward.

"That's not what I meant, I only said it as a way to start a conversation," I replied coolly.

He hadn't been expecting this. He had been expecting me to scurry off. He stared at me from where he was leaning his enormous burly frame back in his chair. The labor and delivery nurses who he had been joking around with at the nurses' station, immediately became quiet. They thrived on drama and did not want to interrupt a possible confrontation. After all, not much else had happened today.

Without taking his eyes off of mine he finally replied, "OK," and heaved himself up from his chair. "Let's go."

The patient was a young woman in her twenties. She had come to the emergency department after experiencing increasing lower abdominal pain. A pregnancy test showed that she was pregnant, however the ultrasound that followed showed that the pregnancy had implanted itself in the wrong part of her uterus. This is what is known as an ectopic pregnancy. Not only can it not be carried forward to birth, but if left untreated it could kill the mother. At this stage, surgery to remove it was the only option.

Dr. Jaggers and I stood in the operating room. The patient was fast asleep, and using a camera, Dr. Jaggers had identified the ectopic pregnancy. "There it is," he announced to no one in particular, conveying his annoyance at having had to get up from his chair to do this surgery. I remember wondering to myself how saving a young lady's life had become so boring to him.

I watched as he excised the ectopic pregnancy from the young lady's right fallopian tube. Afterward, the excision site oozed blood for a bit and he had to dab it with a surgical sponge several times before it stopped. The excision hadn't been sloppy, but it hadn't been particularly elegant either. As soon as the bleeding had finally stopped, Dr. Jaggers remarked, "Good enough." Everyone in the room nodded, and then he closed his incisions, ending the surgery.

Afterward, his words reverberated through my mind, "Good enough." Had he been joking? This woman had entrusted him to do surgery on her, to do the *best* he could to help her, not a mediocre job. "Not only is this guy a dick, but he's also a lazy doctor," I remember thinking to myself.

Near the end of my fourth year of residency I stood in the operating room with my program director Dr. Moore, hunched over a patient on the operating room table. The patient was a man in his thirties who had been in a head-on car crash. Luckily, he had been wearing his seatbelt, the only reason he was still alive. Unluckily, the seatbelt had ruptured a portion of his intestines, something that happens infrequently. I had cut open his abdomen, found the injured bowel, and resected it, as Dr. Moore stood across the table assisting (and silently evaluating) me. She hadn't said a word the entire time. I took the two ends of the uninjured bowel and held them next to each other. They would reconnect just fine.

"Stapler," I said to the scrub tech without taking my eyes off of the bowel. I felt the plastic handle slap into the palm of my left hand, "thank you."

Using it, I reconnected the two ends of bowel making what is known as an anastomosis. When finished, I glanced up at Dr. Moore, trying to read her masked face for any sign of satisfaction or displeasure with my work, but her face was blank like a poker player's. I started to get nervous. If I declared the anastomosis complete, and she did not agree, I risked her thinking I didn't know what I was doing. I glanced up at her face one more time. Still nothing.

I quickly made a decision. "Stitch!" I called to the scrub tech, and immediately felt him slap the metallic handle of the needle driver into my hand. I twisted my wrist, preparing to place the suture when I felt a hand on top of mine, stopping me. I looked up at Dr. Moore who was holding back my hand.

"What are you doing?" she asked me, speaking for the first time.

"It looks like it needs another stitch," I replied, trying to sound confident.

"Why?"

"It could be better."

"Ahhh," she said, knowingly. "Do you know what the enemy of good is?"

"The enemy of what?" I stammered, confused.

"The enemy of good?" she repeated.

By this point in residency, I thought that I knew the answer to every question any attending could ask me. But I did not know the answer to this one.

"No," I replied, feeling my cheeks warm with embarrassment.

"The enemy of good, is better," she said.

Even behind my surgical mask it was obvious that I was still not following. She continued, "Right now this anastomosis is good. It is fine. It will serve its purpose. If you try to make it better by putting in more sutures, driving the needle through it more, you might ruin it. And then we go from having a perfectly fine anastomosis to a problem. Not everything has to be better, sometimes good enough, is good enough."

My mind instantly flashed back to that moment in the O.R. five years earlier during my third year with the OB-GYN surgeon. I understood now. He hadn't been lazy like I had thought. At some point in his career, he had probably learned the exact same lesson that I was learning right now. Maybe he had even learned it in a much harder way, through inadvertently harming a patient while trying to perfect his work.

Surgery is a balance. Most surgeons are control freaks and perfectionists. But in clinical practice, sometimes the only way to be your best is to stare the enemy of good in the face and know when to stand down.

When it comes down to it, surgeons are a little bit deranged. They have to be. They suffer through five years of sleepless, soul-crushing residency to win the prize at the other end; the right, no, *the privilege*, to take fellow human beings to an isolated part of the hospital, put them to sleep, and then cut them with a scalpel. Outside of the operating room, this would be assault. Then, once we have cut them sufficiently, we stick our hands into their open abdomens and root around in their guts, looking for our target: the rudely ruptured appendix, the persistently bleeding spleen, a kinked piece of bowel, or the chronically inflamed gallbladder. Then, we take it out, hold it in our hands, and proclaim our victory. Our intent is always to help the patient, even if it means administering this form of controlled trauma to them. Sometimes patients end up worse off with more pain than when we started. Sometimes they even die. And what does the surgeon, this sick human being, do then? Apologize to the family. Offer condolences. Reflect on what went wrong. Vow to never let it happen again. And then operate again on the next patient.

The practice of medicine is not perfect. It is often likened to an art. As a result, surgery is an imperfect craft that we strive to perform as perfectly as possible. Although we cannot always control the outcome, we can, and do, meticulously control what we can. That being said, surgeons are humans, and mistakes can still occur, sometimes within our control, sometimes not. Mistakes don't just hurt patients, they hurt the surgeon too, who often feels the impact of a complication long after the patient has recovered.

In the spring of my intern year, I had been invited to attend a wedding back in California. Luckily, I was able to finagle the weekend off, as long as I took call the Thursday night beforehand. This worked out for me because I figured I could sleep on the airplane the next day.

Around three a.m., toward the end of my call shift, I admitted an elderly woman named Mrs. Johnson who had developed bleeding in her brain after a fall. This is what is known as an intracranial hemorrhage. The problem with bleeding in the brain, is that it is relatively inaccessible without surgery to stop, since it is hiding behind the skull. When patients have only a small amount of bleeding, the treatment is to monitor them closely and give medications that function as the opposite of blood thinners like aspirin, to encourage their body to stop the bleeding on its own.

All patients who are admitted to the hospital are at risk of developing blood clots in their legs called DVTs. These clots can randomly dislodge and travel to the lungs, causing a pulmonary embolism, which can be fatal. Therefore, it's routine for patients who are admitted to the hospital to be given a medication called Enoxaparin, to thin their blood. It is so routine, in fact, that ordering this medication is part of the process when admitting a patient to the hospital. In the case of brain bleeds, however, this medication should not be given—for obvious reasons.

That morning, when I had been admitting this new patient with an intracranial hemorrhage to the hospital, without realizing it, I had ordered Mrs. Johnson be given Enoxaparin. Once my shift was done and I had signed out my patients to Kyle, I left and went to the airport.

I had just boarded the airplane and was waiting for the pilot to taxi to runway and take off when my phone buzzed. I looked down and saw a text message from Kyle: "Dude, why'd you order Enoxaparin for Mrs. Johnson? She has a brain bleed!!!"

The plane lurched forward, heading toward the runway. "Please turn off all electronic devices including cellphones!" the flight attendant was instructing overhead.

Quickly, I fired off one last text to Kyle, "PLEASE CANCEL THE ORDER!!!"

The entire flight, despite my exhaustion from working the entire night before, I could not sleep. I sat in my chair, terrified, anxiously wondering if I had just killed a patient. I felt sick.

After what felt like an eternity, the plane landed, and I frantically turned on my cellphone. Almost immediately, it buzzed, and I raced to the open the text message from Kyle: "Too late dude, she died."

My heart sank and I wanted to cry. How would I face anyone at work ever again? Would I even still have a job after Dr. Moore found out about this?

My phone buzzed again, and I looked down. Another text message from Kyle. Probably giving me a heads up that I was going to be in a lot of trouble when I got back. Gingerly I opened it: "Just kidding. I cancelled the order before she got the medication. Have fun at the wedding!!!"

I was so relieved that I nearly stood up and started cheering. People on the plane around me would have thought I was insane.

During my third year of residency, I had a thirty-eight-year-old patient, Donna, who had developed thyroid cancer and we had to remove her thyroid. The thyroid is a small gland about the size of half of an apple. It is imbedded on the front of the neck and sits on either side of the trachea, or windpipe, with a small piece that crosses over the front of it. Surgery to remove the thyroid gland is meticulous. It's often a very lengthy surgery, because this area also contains several important nerves and arteries.

The attending surgeon, Dr. Beaumont, and I had been working all day freeing either side of the thyroid gland from Donna's neck. It was now late in the afternoon and one of the final steps left was to remove the part of the gland that crosses over the trachea, called the isthmus.

"Want to do it?" Dr. Beaumont grunted from behind his mask.

"Yes," I said, doing my best to hide any hint of fatigue from my voice.

He grunted again and handed me a tiny pair of extremely sharp scissors.

"Just dissect really slowly and stay off of the trachea."

"Ok, got it."

I placed the tips of the scissors just under the isthmus of the thyroid gland and opened them slowly. I felt very little resistance, which was reassuring. It meant that I was in the right plane. I repeated this gesture several more times, advancing the scissors gently forward each time, slowly separating the gland from the trachea underneath it. It was easier than I had thought it would be. Confidently, I kept pushing forward.

Suddenly, I felt a pop, there was a rush of air, and immediately we smelled the anesthetic gasses escaping from the patient's airway.

"What did I just tell you not to do?" Dr. Beaumont glared at me.

He snatched the scissors away from me, quickly completed the dissection exposing in full view the hole I had created in the patient's trachea.

"Get me some PDS suture," he told the scrub tech.

I watched silently as he repaired the hole, my cheeks burning underneath my mask.

"She'll be fine," he said, once he had finished.

We finished the remainder of the operation without any further issues. Once we had stepped out of the operating room, Dr. Beaumont turned to me and said, "Now we have to go tell the patient's family what happened." I followed him to the waiting room, where Donna's brother and mother had been waiting all day.

We called them into a private consultation room and told them that, overall, the operation had gone fine, that we had been able to remove the entire thyroid gland with the cancer, as planned. They cheered and thanked us.

"But there is something else," he slowly added.

They froze, listening.

"While we were dissecting the middle part of the gland off of the trachea, a hole was made in her trachea," he said, careful not to assign blame.

The patient's mother gasped and clutched her hands to her mouth. After she had composed herself, she asked, "Does this mean that she will have to breathe through a tube for the rest of her life?"

"No, no, no. Nothing like that. I fixed the hole. It should heal fine. Does she still smoke?"

"Yes," came her brother's voice.

"It's now more important than ever that she stop, to help the hole heal."

"Ok, we will let her know," her mother promised.

Donna went home from the hospital the next day without any issues and in good spirits. I breathed a sigh of relief. But that wouldn't be the last time I saw her.

A week later, Donna returned to the emergency department. Earlier that day she had started to feel that her face was puffy. She looked in the mirror, and to her shock and horror, her entire face was swollen from the neck up. When she touched her cheeks, she said they felt crunchy, like bubble wrap. Scared and unsure what was going on, she called 911, and they brought her to the emergency department.

Unbeknownst to her, the hole in her trachea had failed to heal and opened up. Air from her trachea escaped, and trapped underneath her skin, traveled upward, blowing her entire face up like a balloon. Under different circumstances, this might have been funny.

Dr. Beaumont and I privately guessed that she had probably continued to smoke despite our instructions. Either way, it was our fault—more specifically, mine—that a hole in her trachea had occurred in the first place. I felt horrible.

We re-operated, drained the air out of her face, and closed the hole again. She stayed in the hospital for about a week afterward, so we could monitor her progress and ensure that she didn't smoke. This time around, she left the hospital and did not have to return.

All's well that ends well, I thought.

During my fourth year of residency, I had a thirty-two-year-old patient named Juan, a construction worker. He had been admitted to the hospital with abdominal pain. After examining him and reviewing his CT scan, it was clear that his pain was due to an abdominal wall hernia, or weakness in the abdominal wall. A portion of his small bowel had become trapped within the defect. This causes his bowel to become kinked like a garden hose, which in turn caused him severe abdominal pain. He clearly needed surgery.

Before surgery, Juan asked us, "How long will the recovery be? I need to return to work. My wife just had a baby, and she isn't working right now."

"A few days in the hospital, then another week of rest at home. You won't be able to lift anything heavy for two months though," I explained to him. "Does your job offer light duty?" I was trying to put his mind at ease and reassure him that he would still be able to work to support his family while he recovered.

Dr. Stillman and I took Juan to the operating room and opened his abdomen. We carefully examined the piece of bowel that had gotten caught in the hernia.

"What do you want to do, Dr. McPherson?" Dr. Stillman queried me from across the operating table.

"It's dead, I need to remove it," I replied.

"How do you know?" came a voice to my left. It belonged to Mike, an eager third-year medical student.

"Look how pink the rest of the bowel is. That bowel is normal, healthy. Now look at this piece here that I'm holding, it's practically black, dead," I replied patiently.

"How did that happen?"

"When it got caught in the hernia it got kinked. That blocked the little blood vessels that supply it with blood. Without blood, it died."

"Can't you just un-kink it and the vessels will open back up? Do you really need to take it out?"

"The damage has been done. It won't come back to life," I said, beginning to grow impatient. "Dead is dead. If I don't take it out now, it will perforate later and make this man very sick."

"Gotcha," Mike replied.

I worked to remove the one-foot segment of bowel that had died, then reconnected the still-living ends. This restored continuity to the patient's intestinal tract.

"Now, how do you want to close the hernia?" Dr. Stillman asked me, referring to the weakness in the patient's abdominal wall that had caused the problem. There was a myriad of ways to close the defect.

"P-D-S," I replied, sounding out each letter as I said it. PDS is a type of suture that stands for Polydioxanone Suture. Between us residents we called it Perfect Damn Suture because it could be used for almost anything.

"Use Ethibond instead. Figure of eight fashion," he replied.

Ethibond is a braided suture, meaning that several tiny sutures smaller than a human hair had been twisted together like a rope. This makes the tensile strength of the suture very strong. The drawback is that it is more difficult to tie sturdy knots.

"Sure thing."

He watched me place the first few sutures, and satisfied with my technique, he tore off his surgical gown and left Mike and me to finish. Meticulously I placed all of the sutures and then tied all of the knots myself. These sutures and my knots would be responsible for holding the patient's abdomen closed, keeping his intestines safe inside, while our incision healed.

After surgery, the patient was admitted to a room in the hospital where we would monitor him for the next few days while he recovered. Everything went fine until the third day after his operation.

"Dr. McPherson!" came Mike's breathless voice.

"I told you, call me Ryan."

It was six-thirty a.m. I was sitting at a computer reviewing the charts of all of the patients on the list. One of Mike's jobs as a medical student was to round on patients, similar to what residents do.

"I just rounded on Juan Hernandez, something's wrong."

"Oh, really?" I said doubtfully as I opened his chart on the computer in front of me. All of his labs and vital signs were normal.

"I took down the dressing from his abdominal wound like you told me, and a lot of fluid came out!" he exclaimed.

I sat bolt upright in my chair. "What color was the fluid?"

"Pink, like salmon."

"C'mon, let's go!" I replied, hastily grabbing my white coat off the back of my chair as I stood up.

"Sorry to wake you," I said as I turned all of the lights on in Mr. Hernandez's room.

"No problem. Can't really sleep in this place anyways," he replied.

"I need to take a look at your incision."

"No problem," he said, pulling up his hospital gown, exposing a white bandage that was soaked with fluid.

I knelt down at his bedside and gently removed the tape around the edges of the bandage, which was no trouble at all since the fluid had already done most of the work. Once the tape was free, I easily peeled the remainder of the bandage off of his abdomen, exposing the wound underneath. To my dismay, the edges of the wound had come apart. In the middle of the wound the sutures were loose, my unraveled knots the clear culprit. Tying knots is one of the most basic proficiencies in surgery, and I, a senior resident, had messed it up. Worse yet, some of his intestines had begun to poke out through the wound.

I stood up slowly and cleared my throat. "Unfortunately, we are going to need to take you back to the O.R. The wound on your abdomen needs to be re-closed."

"Why, what happened? Did I do something wrong?"

Mike and the patient were both staring at me intently, waiting for my reply. I felt my face flush with embarrassment. "No, err, you didn't do anything wrong. Unfortunately, some of the knots came undone."

"Will I still be able to go back to work in a week like you said before?"

"Unfortunately, no. This will delay your recovery a little bit."

"I see. Well, you have to do what you have to do. I trust you." Hearing these last three words, "I trust you," made me feel worse. It was because he had trusted me that he was in this predicament to begin with.

Dr. Stillman arrived at the hospital at seven a.m. sharp. "Let's round!" He was in good spirits. This was going to make my next task even more difficult.

"Before we begin, I need to tell you something," I said, aware again of Mike watching me. His job as a med student was to shadow residents and learn. He wasn't doing anything wrong, but his presence felt like an audience. At this embarrassing moment, an audience was the last thing I wanted, and I resented him being there.

"What?" Dr. Stillman asked suspiciously.

"You remember Juan Hernandez?"

"Yes."

I paused, wishing time would stop so that I wouldn't have to tell him. So that I could spare myself the embarrassment and his disappointment. Dr. Stillman, you may remember, was not only my boss, but also my friend.

"Yes," he repeated. "Post-operative day 3 ventral hernia repair, right? What about him?"

"The sutures failed, and his wound opened," I said, the words tumbling out of my mouth.

"Are you sure?"

"Yes. The wound is totally open, and his bowel is coming out."

He exhaled and flashed me a look of annoyance. "Ok. Go talk to the O.R. and find out when we can take him back." Then he added, "You're going to fix this."

Secretly, I had been hoping that Dr. Stillman would be so upset with me that he would not allow me to participate in the re-operation. That he would re-close the patient's abdomen on his own, to ensure that it was done properly. But his last words, "You're going to fix this," made me squirm. He was not going to save me. I was far enough along in training that it was now up to me to fix my own mistakes. In the operating room that afternoon, I felt like a race car driver racing on the same track I had crashed and nearly died on, terrified of making the same mistake twice.

The re-operation went fine, and Juan was again admitted to the hospital for observation while he recovered. The next morning, I told Mike not to round on him. I gave him the excuse that Juan had been through enough already and didn't need to be bothered early in the morning. Secretly though, I didn't want anyone else to see the results of my work until I was certain the re-operation had been successful. I didn't think I could tolerate another failure.

I stood inside Juan's room, alone, and examined his abdomen. Everything looked fine. I breathed a sigh of relief.

"Again, I'm sorry this happened. I know you need to get back to work and this has been a setback for you and your new family."

"It's ok. These things happen," he said.

I was shocked at his calm and non-accusatory demeanor. I had expected him to be upset with me. I've seen customers at Starbucks lose their minds over getting the wrong kind of milk in their latte. But he didn't react that way at all. I admired him for that.

CHAPTER 19—M&M

I f a resident was party to a mistake in caring for a surgical patient, they were reprimanded. This took the form of appearing at a *Morbidity and Mortality Conference*, which everyone calls M&M. M&M is a form of peer review that is meant to put the mistake(s) under a proverbial microscope, discuss the mistake(s), identify why it happened and decide what can be done to prevent it from happening again. Every M&M conference would begin with the reminder, "We take care of over 3,000 patients per year. We are only going to be discussing the few in which things went wrong. If we sat around all day discussing all the ones which we did a good job, we wouldn't learn anything."

Not so bad, right?

The thing about M&M is that it can feel humiliating. In the setting of a formal weekly conference, you stand before all of your co-residents while attending surgeons ask you questions, picking apart the case that you were involved in that went awry. These questions are crafted, almost as if by a lawyer, in a way that makes you contradict yourself and exposes the flaws in your thinking ... in front of everyone else.

Despite years of training and education, whenever I presented at M&M, I was reduced to feeling like I did early in my intern year trying to find help for the lady feigning a pseudo seizure. Here's an example:

"Dr. McPherson, when evaluating this young lady in the emergency room for abdominal pain did you consider appendicitis may be the cause?"

"Yes."

"But you didn't think she had appendicitis?"

"Correct."

"Do you know how to diagnose appendicitis?"

"Yes, of course."

"Then why didn't you think she had appendicitis?"

"Well, her abdomen was pretty benign when I examined her—"

"Did you examine her or the medical student?"

"I did!"

"Ok. Interesting, because when I examined her later, her abdomen was definitely not 'benign.'"

"Well, also her labs and CT scan were equivocal …"

"Did you look at the CT scan yourself or just read what the radiologist wrote?"

"I looked at it."

"Are you sure?"

"Yes."

"Ok, let's review the CT scan here together." The CT scan would then be projected onto a large screen for everyone to see. "Dr. McPherson, do me a favor and point to the appendix so we can all see it."

Pointing at the appendix, "Here."

"And you think that doesn't look like appendicitis?"

"Well, I thought it could be an early appendicitis."

"Ok, fine, I'll give you that. Even though you just told me that YOU thought she had a benign abdomen and that YOU didn't think she had appendicitis. Then tell me this, if YOU weren't sure whether or not she had appendicitis, then why did you start antibiotics, why didn't you observe her off of antibiotics and let the appendicitis declare itself?"

"Err," I stammered. By now it was clear to everyone I had made a mistake.

"Don't you realize that starting antibiotics could have mask the early signs of appendicitis making achieving the correct diagnosis even more unlikely?"

"Err … well, like I said, I thought she had an early appendicitis and I wanted to start treating her."

"First you tell me she didn't have appendicitis, and then you think she may have had an early appendicitis and you want to treat her with antibiotics

... You're losing me here ..."

"I thought she may have an early appendicitis."

"OK, GREAT! But what's the treatment for appendicitis in a young healthy patient? Is it antibiotics and observe them?"

"No, typically we offer surgery."

"Then why not take her to the operating room and do ... SURGERY?!"
Silence.

"Wait, I know. Please tell me you offered her surgery and that she refused, and that's why you decided to admit her and treat her appendicitis with antibiotics instead. Is that what happened?"

"No, she didn't refuse surgery. I was still unsure if she had appendicitis or not and I did not want to subject her to an unnecessary operation."

"Do you know what I found the next day when I operated on her?"

"Yes."

"What did I find, tell me."

"You found a gangrenous appendicitis."

"Exactly. Do you think that I subjected her to an 'unnecessary' operation?"

"No."

"No, of course not. I found a nearly perforated appendix. It was gangrenous. Ready to burst. You missed the diagnosis. Her labs, CT scan, and physical exam were anything but equivocal. I'm not even convinced you ever saw the patient. You delayed treatment. If you had caused us to wait any longer, her appendix would have perforated, and she would have needed an even bigger operation. Is that what you wanted to happen?"

"No, of course not." My cheeks burned.

"This is a SURGICAL residency program. What do you think we are trying to teach you to do? Not to operate on people who need operations?"

"Well, no, but I wasn't sure if —"

"Sit down. Let the next resident come up here and present, unless it's you again. God, I hope it's not you again."

Despite the embarrassment, (not only for myself, but also when my co-residents were presenting) I found these weekly conferences to be a veritable Mecca of education. If I wasn't the one presenting, I would sit, paralyzed, while I watched my fellow residents undergo the needling questions. First, they'd squirm, then they'd try to retract things they said, and eventually they succumbed to the fact that they had made a mistake. While watching, I would squirm with them, and feel what they were feeling, listening intently, imaging how it could have just as easily been me up there.

It feels terrible to have your mistakes openly discussed and criticized. M&M has a purpose, though. Through this discomfort, learning occurs. M&M provides a forum to learn from your own mistakes, as well as the mistakes of others. By the time myself or one of my co-residents finished presenting, *I* felt defeated, embarrassed, even though I had only been watching. But as a result of this emotional toll, I learned how to avoid the mistakes that had been discussed. Each mistake presented in M&M was seared into my mind like a cattle brand, and I am proud to say that I never repeated a mistake that anyone had ever presented in M&M.

M&M doesn't end with residency. At most institutions M&M continues even for attending surgeons. M&M is a tradition unique to surgery; it isn't practiced by other medical specialties. This is probably due to the invasive nature of surgery and the fact that surgeons pride themselves on always trying to do better. When you boil down to it, surgery is intentionally inflicting trauma onto a fellow human being in an attempt to improve them in some way. That improvement might be relieving pain, curing cancer, or stopping bleeding. Surgery is inherently dangerous and rife with potential complications.

Prescribing medications to patients is much less dangerous. When a patient makes their way through the health care system, many things will happen. If, during that time, a physician prescribes the incorrect drug to a patient, it *rarely* results in immediate complications, and is therefore much harder for patients to pinpoint as the exact cause of their ongoing suffering.

Surgery, on the other hand, is much easier to identify as a 'sentinel event' that led to their decline. "Before surgery I had reflux, but since surgery, I have constant abdominal pain, trouble swallowing, and can no longer eat my favorite foods …"

Surgeons are constantly concerned about complications, because of the catastrophic effects they can have on patient's lives. Complications oftentimes don't kill patients, but they can sometimes leave patients disabled or with intractable pain, wishing that they had died instead. Sometimes complications are inevitable, a byproduct of the circumstances in which the surgery had to be done. An example would be a trauma patient who has been shot in the abdomen, and the bullet punctures their colon. This causes them to leak stool all over the inside of their abdomen. These patients are more likely to get a wound infection than, say, someone undergoing an elective hernia repair—regardless of the surgeon's skill.

When complications happen, the surgeon feels responsible and will do everything within their ability to right the wrong. Every surgeon knows numerous stories of complications that have happened to patients, by their own hands, or the hand of other surgeons. When complications happen, the patient and the surgeon both suffer, though in different ways.

Countless surgeons have lost countless hours of sleep because they've laid awake at night, replaying every decision they made, every move they made in the O.R., and figuring out what they could do differently to prevent another complication from happening. Complications weigh heavily on surgeons' minds, each one like a cut that leaves a scar.

CHAPTER 20—The Prisoner

The tail end of my fifth and final year of residency, which is also known as "chief year," happened in 2020 and coincided with COVID-19's arrival in the United States. Initially, hospitals continued business as normal. But as word spread that hospitals in Italy, and soon after, New York, were becoming overwhelmed, it became clear that more would have to be done.

Some of the first measures introduced at our hospital were: screening all employees for fevers and symptoms before entering, wearing masks, not allowing visitors, and cancelling all non-emergency surgeries. As a result, my final months of residency were spent performing exclusively urgent surgeries. It was also during this time that Dr. Stillman let me perform an entire carotid endarterectomy—a delicate procedure to remove plaque from the main blood vessel in the neck—for the first time. I had never heard of him letting any of the residents do an *entire* carotid endarterectomy before.

The carotid artery supplies the brain with blood. After a certain point, built-up plaque becomes dangerous and increases the risk of stroke. To remove the plaque, the artery needs to be dissected in the patient's neck, opened, the plaque removed using a fine instrument called a *scraper*, and the vessel re-closed. All without starving the brain of blood. Each of these steps must be performed swiftly and perfectly, otherwise the risk increases that the patient will have a stroke during the surgery.

I had assisted Dr. Stillman with a number of these surgeries before and I knew how particular he was about each step, each movement, the way

179

each piece of tissue was handled. At times it could be downright frustrating, because he was so *particular*. As a result, though, his operations were speedy, and he had excellent outcomes. For these reasons, I know he would not have let me do the operation unless he believed I was ready. I finally began to feel like I was becoming a competent surgeon.

The patient, Mr. Granger, was a gangly seventy-nine-year-old Caucasian man who looked twenty years younger. He had short white hair that stuck up in all different directions, and a matching white beard. He smiled frequently, revealing a few missing teeth. He was a pleasant guy. He had been brought to the hospital after having a T.I.A.

T.I.A. is short for *transient ischemic attack*, which is often described as being a "mini stroke" because all of the symptoms of the stroke resolve within twenty-four hours. It is a notable occurrence, because it serves as a warning that a real stroke is coming soon. A T.I.A. is usually the result of plaque build-up in one of the carotid arteries. When we did an ultrasound of Mr. Granger's carotid artery, that was exactly what we found. In fact, his plaque build-up was so significant that it was occluding over 90% of his artery, which allowed only a small amount of blood to get to his brain. What made Mr. Granger different, however, was the presence of two big burly men seated at his bedside. They were both federal prison officers, there to ensure Mr. Granger didn't make a break for it, or worse, that he didn't attack anyone.

This was not the first time that I had cared for a prisoner. The first time I had to do so was in med school. I had been sent into a patient's room alone to interview and examine him. Mid-examination, I discovered he was handcuffed to the bed. At that moment I realized the two police officers at his bedside were not his friends. At first, the experience was unnerving. I'd seen plenty of movies that portrayed prisoners as caged lions, always dangerous. While I do recommend keeping your guard up, after taking care of a number of prisoners, I discovered that they were actually great patients. They were generally polite and grateful for the care we took of them. This is because being in the hospital, normally a nightmare for most people, can be like a vacation for them.

I interviewed Mr. Granger to learn more about his scant medical history. I asked him about other stroke symptoms he might have had. Next, I explained that one of the main arteries in his neck responsible for providing the brain with blood was over 90% narrowed, and that we would need to do surgery to fix it. He was eager to talk and kept me there as long as he could, asking me questions about everything. Just when I was about to leave, he would think of another 'medical' question to ask. I imagined that he was probably lonely. I doubted that his guards were interested in talking to him.

Eventually, I summed up everything that we had talked about and asked—for the *fifth* time—if he had any more questions. He paused, glanced up toward the ceiling deep in thought, and finally unable to think of another question, shrugged, and said, "I guess you have to do what you have to do."

I turned to the guards. I knew that they would also have questions. Theirs, however, had nothing to do with medicine or the surgery we were planning to perform. They were merely interested in logistics. They wanted to know when the surgery would be performed and how long he would have to stay in the hospital afterward. By the time I had finished answering their questions, Mr. Granger had thought of one more question. "When you are through with surgery, can you call my sister and let her know how I am doing?"

I glanced over at the guards who both shook their heads. After seeing this, I turned back at the patient and verbally re-iterated what the guard's body language had clearly told me, "No, I am sorry, I won't be able to call her."

Updating a patient's family after surgery is routine. I was both surprised and unsure why the guards had nixed it so quickly. Later, when I was speaking to a colleague, I found out that it was for security purposes. No one in the outside world could know the prisoner-patient was temporarily in a hospital, let alone *which* hospital, because there was a chance they'd come and try to free him. Still, I felt bad not being able to share with his family that he was having urgent surgery.

In the US, when people go to jail, the results of their trial and why they are in jail become public records, easily searchable by anyone. During the times that I have taken care of inmates as patients, I have always made it a habit of treating them the exact same way as I would any other patient. To me, part of doing so, is not attempting to learn any more about them than what they have told me. This includes not looking up their name on the internet. It's not just that I view it as a form of respect (which I do), but I simply don't ever want to take the risk that I might allow their crimes to (subconsciously) cloud my clinical judgement. Some of my colleagues, on the other hand, didn't feel the same way.

Once in the operating room it was business as usual. The anesthesiologist, Dr. Abebe, used the same line he used every time he administered anesthesia, "Pick out a nice dream!"

The only difference was the presence of our guest, one of the prison guards. Per some policy somewhere, at least one prison guard had to remain with the patient at all times. I wondered what had happened in the past that had resulted in such a policy. Had a prisoner suddenly woken up from deep anesthesia and fled the hospital mid operation with a gaping wound in his neck? I guess you can never be too careful. In any case, I had an additional spectator that day.

The split-second the patient was asleep, the gossip began. Dr. Abebe looked up and excitedly asked Dr. Stillman and I over the surgical drapes, "Did you hear what this guy did!?"

I ignored him. This was an advanced surgery, and I was focused on making the perfect incision. Dr. Stillman, also ignoring him, was watching me like a hawk. I was determined not to give Dr. Stillman even the slightest reason to take the operation away from me.

Unencumbered and eager to engage, Joey, my junior resident who was standing next to me blurted out, "Yeah! I just read about it online."

I felt the patient's skin open as I slid the scalpel along his neck, doing my best to ignore the chatter around me.

"He's as good as a killer. That's why they've got him in for life," came the guard's voice from the corner of the room.

"Apparently, Mr. Granger here has been in jail for thirty years!" came Dr. Abebe's voice, his head still craning over the surgical drapes.

"Yup," the guard grunted. "Thirty years, at least."

"I read he hired a hitman to kill his brother," Joey was saying.

"That's right!" Dr. Abebe interjected. "Even though he had already made millions of dollars on his own, he wanted to cut his brother out of some sort of inheritance or something."

From the corner of the room, "Greedy, he wanted even more money. Tell you what, if I had a couple million dollars, I would be quiet as a clam."

Following this was a collective "Mmm hmm" from nearly every person in the room.

I was trying hard to ignore them, hoping they would move on to something else. But instead, the story continued.

"Apparently the hitman, Ron, was not so good," Dr. Abebe continued. "According to the news article I read, one weekday morning Ron dressed up as a postal delivery man and went to the brother's house and rang the doorbell." He was speaking animatedly, and from the corner of my eyes I could see he was gesturing with his hands, acting out the entire scene. Anesthesiologists really only need to pay attention to the patient when they are going to sleep and when they are waking up, freeing them up to socialize while the surgeons are working.

He waved his arms around as he continued, "When the brother answered the door, Ron asked him to sign for a package. When he had finished signing, the brother asked where the package was and Ron hit him in the face with his gun, knocking him unconscious. And then this is where things get really ugly." He paused to catch his breath. "That's when Ron pulled the unconscious brother into the house, so that he could do the deed in private instead of on the guy's front lawn. But that's when he realized that the brother's wife and son were still home and had seen him! Not wanting to leave behind any witnesses, he decided to murder them as well. While he was doing this, the brother woke up and escaped from the house. Bleeding from his face, he ran across the street to an elementary school, searching for help. Apparently, it was the middle of recess or something and Ron decided not to follow him into the school yard and finish the job, so he bailed. Obviously, the police caught this chucklehead almost right away," Dr. Abebe said, wrapping up the story. "Can you believe that!?"

"There are some real psychos out there," came the guard's voice.

Gaining his second wind, Dr. Abebe continued again, "Once the police got him, Ron immediately turned on Mr. Granger, who of course was then sentenced to life in jail. According to the court records, Granger pled not guilty."

"He still denies it to this day," came the guard's voice again.

By now I was halfway through with the operation. I had exposed the carotid artery, opened it, and was nearly done removing the plague from it. Dr. Stillman had continued to watch me quietly the entire time. Finally, the conversation moved on.

"Is your job like in the movies?" Dr. Abebe was asking the guard. This was ironic because normally we are the ones being asked if our job is like *Grey's Anatomy*.

"Well," the guard replied, thinking, "like, which movie?"

"*Shawshank Redemption*," Joey blurted out.

"Yeah! *Shawshank Redemption*. I bet it's at least a little bit like that!" came Dr. Abebe's animated voice.

Chuckling, the guard replied, "No, not really. That's just a movie. But we do move the prisoners' rooms around every so often to prevent them from being able to pull off anything like they did in that movie, you know, how they slowly dug that hole to escape through."

Since this was a dead end, Dr. Abebe changed the subject again, "How have you guys been dealing with COVID in the jails?"

"Well, for one, we aren't taking any new prisoners. Instead, the county jails are becoming overcrowded holding people, and even letting criminals out. We've also been requiring all prisoners to wear masks. The problem with the masks though is that the part that fits around the nose has a small piece of metal in it. The prisoners are smart and have figured out that they can take this piece of metal out and use it to escape from their hand cuffs."

"No kidding!"

"Yeah, here, let me show you."

This, I was interested in. I stopped operating and looked up so that I could watch along with the rest of the room as the guard showed us precisely how to escape from handcuffs with nothing more than a small fragment of metal.

Then he added, "It can be scary. Sometimes they take them off because they want to fight you. Other times they just hand them back to you and laugh because they think it's funny."

I imagined the sheer terror that would rush through me if I were a guard and a prisoner did this to me.

As I put in the final stitches, closing the incision on the patient's neck that I had made less than ninety minutes earlier, I said "Yo, Abebe! We are done here, wake him up!"

Dr. Abebe's head popped over the drapes and he stared down at my hands, checking to make sure I was really done before waking the patient up. He said, "Wow, that was fast," and then he started busily turning knobs and dials. Conversation halted and the room grew quiet as the patient woke up.

The surgery had gone well. The steps of the procedure that I normally watched Dr. Stillman do, had proved to me more difficult than I had anticipated. But under his constant watchful eye, despite the conversation in the room, my focus had been unshakable, my hands steady. I finally started to feel like the thousands of hours of training were beginning to pay off.

CHAPTER 21—The Worst Color in Medicine

I was driving home late on a Wednesday afternoon near the end of my chief year. I had less than two months to go before graduation. In my kitchen hung a calendar that I marked off daily, counting down to graduation. When I got home, I was going to place a large "X" through today's date.

Traffic was heavy, and it was raining, so I hadn't made it very far before Gabby, the junior resident on call, called and told me that the emergency department had just admitted a patient with a possible case of *necrotizing fasciitis* ("flesh eating bacteria"). This was a surgical emergency, if it truly was necrotizing fasciitis.

I didn't want to be liable for having missed such a treacherous diagnosis. I hung up, exhaled, and made my way back to the hospital. One of these days, I would get to leave work without having to go right back, but for now, the "X" on my calendar would have to wait.

Back at the hospital, I walked through the emergency department in search of the alleged necrotizing fasciitis patient's room. As I rounded a corner, I bumped into one of the emergency medicine nurses who told me I was about to get consulted on another patient as well. "Butt puss," she said with a smirk.

"Great, thanks," I said dryly, thinking back to my first encounter in medical school. I already had an idea what kind of a night it was going to be.

186

I evaluated the patient with alleged necrotizing fasciitis and determined that it was nothing more than simple cellulitis, a bacterial infection of the skin. The patient would be fine with some antibiotics. I could put away my scalpel for now. Patients always laugh when I say this last part.

Next, Gabby and I went to go see the "butt puss" patient. Perirectal abscesses can cause a huge amount of discomfort and make patients very sick, but treating them is not glamorous, as you may have noticed at the beginning of this book. It is not unheard of for medical students and O.R. staff to vomit during the operation.

Gabby and I walked into the patient's room. Lying on his side on the gurney in front of us was a forty-five-year-old overweight Hispanic man named Jesus. He had a history of asthma and diabetes. He had come to the hospital because he had been having pain that prevented him from being able to sit. He only spoke Spanish, so Gabby translated as he told us about his symptoms.

"He started having pain about four days ago," she translated. "He is saying that last night he started having fevers and today the pain is much worse."

I nodded along so Jesus could see I understood what she was saying.

"Ok, tell him we have to take a look, he can stay how he is lying on his side. It will just take a minute," I said to her, which she said to him.

Gabby and I examined the area that was causing him pain and agreed that there was definitely an abscess. It wasn't a life-or-death situation, but it was causing him pain, and we were already there, so I decided that we should drain it that evening.

The patient said something in Spanish. "What's he saying?" I asked Gabby.

"He is asking why this happened to him."

"A combination of his diabetes and bad luck. Tell him we have to cut it open and ask him if he wants us to do it with him awake or asleep."

"Asleep!" he nearly shouted, the second the last part left her mouth.

I flashed a thumbs up at him and in return he thanked me saying, "Gracias, gracias" and placed his hands together as if in prayer.

I stepped outside and dialed the phone number for the O.R. front desk. They were not going to like this.

"O.R. front desk, this is Katie speaking."

"Katie, it's Ryan McPherson, I need to add one on."

"Ok, what've you got?"

"Perirectal abscess."

"Butt puss! Are you serious? We all just had dinner, can't you go find something good instead?" she said half-jokingly.

"What are you talking about? This is good! It's quick, we'll be done in five minutes," I said, trying to placate her.

"Fine! I'll get the room set up now."

Despite how unappealing the surgery could be, at least the operation was quick. Hopefully I would be home soon to cross out the "X" of another day.

Within thirty minutes, Gabby, Dr. Abebe the anesthesiologist, and I were all standing in the O.R., helping Jesus move from the hospital gurney onto the firm black operating room table. Lying on his back on the table he grimaced.

"Don't worry you'll be asleep soon," Dr. Abebe said in English. Then realizing his mistake, he said to Gabby, "Tell him he will feel better in a minute once he's asleep."

As she repeated this to him in Spanish, Dr. Abebe placed an oxygen mask over Jesus's face and added, "and tell him to pick out a nice dream," and with that he injected a syringe full of the milky white medication propofol into the patient's IV, putting him to sleep.

After Jesus was asleep, the Dr. Abebe attempted to insert a breathing tube through the patient's mouth and into his windpipe. This would allow Jesus to be connected to a ventilator that would breathe for him while he was under. While I waited, I stood off to the side of the room and scrolled through Instagram on my phone. 99.999% of the time this tube insertion is routine and without issue. This, however, was the 0.001% of the time.

From the corner of my eye, I could see that something wasn't right. I put my phone away and looked up. Dr. Abebe was moving around frantically grabbing at several items and twisting various knobs on the anesthesia machine. I noticed a look of panic on his face. Remember before when I told you that the anesthesiologist's job mostly takes place when the patient

188

is going to sleep and when they are waking up? This is why.

"Everything okay?" I asked.

"Not quite," came the response.

I quickly walked over to the patient's left side to try and get a better idea of exactly what was going on.

"He's asleep and I can't get the tube in," Dr. Abebe said between hurried movements of his arms. "He's in laryngospasm!"

"Ok, just bag him then," I said, referring to using a balloon-shaped bag called an "Ambu bag" to blow air through the patient's mouth and supply his lungs with oxygen.

"I tried already," he said putting the Ambu bag over the patient's mouth. "But his throat is all closed up, see. What's his sat?"

I looked up at the monitor, "88%," I reported back. The patient's oxygen saturation level had fallen from 100%. Eighty-eight percent was not good, but it wasn't deadly either.

"Shit. I'm going to try to look again," Dr. Abebe said, pulling the Ambu bag off of the patient's face. He inserted a metal blade that looks like a small sword into the patient's mouth. This is called a laryngoscope and helps open up the back of the throat to help see while placing the breathing tube. The longer he had the blade in the patient's mouth without giving him oxygen, the less oxygen the patient had in his blood. I eyed the monitor closely.

"We are down to 75%," I said, a sense of urgency growing in my voice. "Do you think you can get it in?"

"No!" came the frantic response. "Let's try to bag him again."

I squeezed the bag hard while he held it tight against the patient's mouth with both hands. We both stared at the monitor hoping the oxygen saturation would increase, but it only continued to fall. We were having an airway emergency. It is rare for patients to die during anesthesia in the twenty-first century, but this was exactly one of the ways it can still happen. In fact, this is how comedian Joan Rivers died in 2014. What had only moments ago been a somewhat *funny* surgery had now become a life-or-death emergency.

The oximeter began to alarm as the saturation continued to drop. His oxygen level was now dangerously low, in the 60%s, falling rapidly with each passing second. Before I knew it the machine was reading in the 50%s. I looked down and noticed that the patient's lips had turned blue. This was a sign that his body was becoming starved of oxygen. A bad sign.

Dr. Abebe tried again, frantically, to look with the laryngoscope and place the breathing tube, but he was still unable to. He had run out of things to try. It had been several minutes since Jesus had last had oxygen in his lungs, and it would only take a few more minutes before he would be dead. What we were doing was not working. If one of us didn't do something right now, Jesus was going to die in front of us.

This realization hit me like basketball in the face. Because all Dr. Abebe's efforts were failing, I needed to do something.

"I'm going to cut him!" I yelled.

"Do it! Do it!" Dr. Abebe yelled back as he continued—fruitlessly—trying to place the breathing tube.

I hadn't donned any of my surgical attire yet, and my hands were covered with only loose-fitting generic thin latex gloves that weren't designed for surgery. I was even still wearing my watch.

"Give me the scalpel!" I called out to the scrub tech who rushed over. I was staring down at the front of Jesus's neck deciding where to cut when I felt the scalpel handle being placed into my outstretched hand. What I was going to do was cut the front of Jesus's neck and keep going until I found his trachea. That way I could make a hole it in and insert the breathing tube directly into that hole, bypassing the area in his throat that had closed up. Because of his size, Jesus had a big neck. There was no telling where his trachea was hiding. Complicating things further, I had never done this procedure before. It's very uncommon to ever have to. But I had read about it and rehearsed each step in my mind over and over again, in case I was ever in exactly this situation.

With my right hand, I lifted up Jesus's chin to stretch his neck, trying to smooth out the extra rolls of tissue so that I could decide where to cut. With my left hand (I am left-handed. Yes, left-handed people can become surgeons too!), I placed the sharp edge of the scalpel in the center of the front of his neck, and drug it downward toward his chest, making a vertical incision. I ended up making a longer incision that I would have liked to. But now was not the time to worry about scars. If he lived to get a scar, he would be lucky.

My first incision had severed a vein hiding just underneath the skin and the wound immediately welled up with blood, obscuring the entire surgical field, making it impossible for me to see. This was a bad start. A very bad start.

Regardless, I pressed on. Since I couldn't see, I would have to take a leap of faith and find his trachea by feel. This was especially challenging since the patient had an unusually large neck and his trachea was buried deeper than normal.

I placed my fingers into the pool of blood, hoping to get lucky and feel the trachea at my fingertips, but I didn't. I could tell that I was still several layers away from it. Panic began to sweep over me. The struggle Dr. Abebe had been having placing the breathing tube had initially been *his* problem. The second I got involved and made the patient bleed, I had converted it into *my* problem. Now, not only was he starving for air, but he was bleeding. My mind was racing. Had I just made things worse instead of better?

I glanced up at the patient's face, hoping against hope to see that Dr. Abebe had been able to place the breathing tube while I had been struggling, but just like before, no luck. I was running out of ideas. I feared that I'd made the wrong call and was in the process of helping to kill someone.

By now, things had gone from bad to terrible. When I glanced up at the patient's face, I noticed something else as well; the patient was no longer blue. Instead, he had turned the worst color in medicine: grey. Grey is the opposite of the color pink, the color of life. Grey is the color of death. It is the color of babies who are stillborn. The color of the faces of corpses before the funeral home applies makeup. And now, it was the color of my patient, who I had just assaulted with a scalpel.

An hour ago, this man had walked into the ER, shaken our hands, and thanked me for promising to help him. We had joked with him and told him he would be able to eat dinner as soon as we were done. How had things gone so wrong?

I couldn't imagine any way he could be anything but dead. This was the worst feeling I had ever experienced in my entire life. My entire body was numb. I had not helped fix this young man; I had helped to kill him. I stared at his lifeless grey face for what felt like an eternity.

My old paranoia dominated my brain, momentarily stealing my focus. A ghoulish voice inside my head was laughing and taunting me, *He's going to die because you can't save him! You're not good enough. You never were! That's why no medical schools wanted to take you in the first place, it's a mistake you're even here! Your best contribution to medicine would have been quitting when you had the chance! HA, HA, HA!*

Then, a funny thing happened. By accepting that the patient was dead, I removed the immense pressure of having to successfully complete the procedure. At this point, there was no way I could make things any worse. I boldly re-inserted the finger of my right hand into the inky pool of blood that had filled the gaping hole in his neck and probed into the bottom of the wound. I pretended that I had x-ray vision and imagined each layer of the neck as I used my fingers to guide the blade of the scalpel, blindly transecting each one, making my incision deeper and deeper. My hands and the scalpel were completely submerged in the patient's neck.

I felt all of my senses shut off as all of as my attention focused entirely on my fingertips, giving them a sort of super sensation allowing me to feel what I could not see. I anxiously felt around for the distinctive firm rings of the outer layer of the trachea. The blinding lights and noise of the operating room had long disappeared. I kept cutting and feeling, cutting and feeling, cutting and feeling...

Suddenly, the tip of my right index finger nudged up against something hard, the tracheal ring I had been searching for! It happened so abruptly I couldn't believe it. I felt ecstatic, as like I had just struck gold. I grasped it between my index finger and thumb just to be sure. A surge of hope rushed through me. With my fingers on either side of the rigid hollow trachea, I held it steady. Still unable to see because of the blood, I pushed the scalpel between my two fingers by feel alone, knowing that the trachea was there, held firmly in place by my fingers. Now all I had left to do was use the blade to make a hole in the front of the trachea and insert the breathing tube.

Almost there ... I thought.

Then, as I tried to force the tip of the scalpel into the trachea, the blade snapped in half. I had never had this happen before. I felt like I was just shy of the finish line, and my shoe had become untied, causing me to trip and fall. If what was going on had not been such an emergency, I probably would have made a joke about hospital administration buying the cheap scalpels to save money.

Unbelievable. I can't catch a break with this guy, I thought, as I continued to work despite the broken scalpel blade floating around in the pool of blood where my fingers were.

The scrub tech had seen what had happened and already had another scalpel ready, which he slapped firmly into my hand. Using the new scalpel, I picked up where I had left off. I would have to find the broken scalpel blade later, hopefully not sticking out of one of my fingers.

Finally, with the new blade I was able to make a hole in the windpipe.

"Give me the breathing tube!" I nearly screamed at Dr. Abebe, adrenaline coursing through my entire body.

With a shaking hand he held it out in front of my face. I grabbed it and pushed it into the hole as if it was now *my* life that depended on it.

Dr. Abebe hooked the tube up to the ventilator and began giving the patient rapid breaths. As he did so, I quickly felt around inside the bloody wound and found the broken half of the scalpel blade. I carefully pulled it out, relieved I had not gotten stuck by it.

I pulled my blood-soaked hands out of the patient's neck and stepped back. My gloves hard torn long ago. My hands, watch, and forearms were covered in blood. I felt like I was waking up from a vivid nightmare. As my senses returned, I heard Dr. Abebe saying "Sats are coming up! 80 ... 90 ... 100!"

I looked around. For the first time I noticed how crowded the room had become. The operating room doors were still swinging as even more people ran in. Nurses and anesthesiologists from other O.R.s had rushed to come try to help. There was a line of med students standing against the wall, watching. The on-call trauma surgeon had just stepped in, with her team of residents in tow. Everyone was staring at me standing next to the patient, both of us covered in blood. I looked as though I'd just been caught committing a murder.

I looked back at the patient's face and noticed his color had improved. Like a chameleon, his face had changed from grey, to blue, to a healthy pink. Despite this seemingly good sign, I still felt horrible. Even if his body had survived, it was likely that his brain had died from being without oxygen for so long. It felt like I had been working on his neck for fifteen minutes. Fifteen minutes was too long. We wouldn't know if he was brain dead until the anesthetic wore off.

I walked out of the operating room and spent a while washing Jesus's blood from my hands and arms. As I did this, the patient was taken to the intensive care unit where we would wait and see if he would wake up.

A nurse came up to me and told me the patient's brother was waiting in the waiting room.

"Does he know what happened?" I asked, turning abruptly to face her.

"No. Just that the patient had surgery."

"I will go talk to him," I said, not looking forward to what was next.

As soon as I finished washing my hands I called the hospital's Spanish interpreter, Justina, and asked her to help me speak with the patient's brother. Now that things had gone downhill, I didn't want to put Gabby in the awkward position of having to translate what had just happened. The interpreter met me outside of the O.R. and followed me into the waiting room— which was empty this late at night, except for one person—the patient's brother. He was still wearing his work clothes and looked tired. He stood up the moment I entered the room. I went over to him and sat down, gesturing for him to do the same.

Now was not the time to mince words. I looked him in the eye and after I introduced myself, I told him that there had been a problem.

"I am sorry, I do not have good news," I said, and waited for my words to be translated. I watched his face as Justina repeated my words exactly, his face rapidly changing from a look of fatigue to one of panic.

"*Qué sucedió?!*" he asked frantically, his eyes darting between Justina's face and mine. Justina turned to me, "He is asking what happened?"

"While the anesthesiologist was putting him to sleep for the procedure, his throat closed up and the breathing tube could not be placed. Because of this he went for several minutes without breathing. To try to save his life I cut a hole in the front of his neck called a tracheostomy."

I listened as my words were transformed once again into Spanish. When I heard Justina say "*traqueotomía*," I knew she was nearly finished, and I waited patiently knowing that an onslaught of questions would follow.

"He is asking why this happened," came Justina's voice. They were both looking at me now.

"I spoke with the anesthesiologist, and he thinks that because of your brother's asthma he had a bad reaction to some of the anesthetic gases that he was using to help put him to sleep, and this may have been what caused his throat to close up."

"Is my brother going to be OK?" Justina said, repeating the patient's question in English.

"He is alive," I paused to allow this to be translated, immediately adding, "but unfortunately since he was without oxygen for so long, we don't know yet how his brain will be, we won't know until the anesthetic completely wears off."

"How long will that take?" Justina translated. Even though I could not understand his words when he said them, I could hear his voice growing desperate, like so many patients' family members before him when I'd had to give bad news.

"Not long."

"He is asking if he can see him."

"Yes, of course," I said, standing up and motioning for them to follow.

Throughout residency I had been tasked with giving family members bad news plenty of times. At the time, it had been painful, but now, compared to this, it had been easy. The reality was, most patients who died had been doomed since before they arrived at the hospital. I wasn't responsible for them dying. I hadn't been the person who shot, stabbed, or crashed a car into them. I hadn't perforated their appendix, ruptured their spleen, or given them cancer.

But this was different. I had been involved in what had happened every single step of the way. I had been the one that caved and decided to do the procedure with Jesus asleep. I could have easily done it with him awake, but it would have been much more uncomfortable for him. I had authorized him being brought to the operating room. I had been the one who cut his neck, making him bleed, and then I'd been too slow getting the breathing tube in.

In my mind, my actions were indistinguishable from those of someone pointing a loaded gun at Jesus's head and pulling the trigger.

Overcome with guilt, I had run out of things to say to Jesus's brother as I led him to the intensive care unit where Jesus had been taken. We arrived at Jesus's bedside where he lay motionlessly with the breathing tube protruding from the front of his neck, the quiet whooshing sound of the ventilator breathing for him. His brother grabbed his hand and started to cry.

"Anything yet?" I asked the intensive care nurse who had been assigned to him.

"No, he hasn't moved yet."

I walked away and sat down at the nurses' station. I started mindlessly doing paperwork to distract myself while I waited. Best case scenario, Jesus would wake up and be normal. Worst case scenario, he had become a vegetable and would forever be reliant on life support to remain purposelessly alive.

I was having a hard time focusing and wished I was anywhere else, doing anything else. *Why didn't I quit surgery before when I had the chance?*

One of the medical students who had been in the O.R. came over and quietly sat down near me. He didn't say anything—he assumed I was busy—but he kept glancing over at me. I could sense that he was bursting with questions and wanted to talk about what had just happened. I remembered when I had been in his shoes five *long* years ago, how curious I had been about everything.

"What's up?" I asked, acknowledging his presence without looking up.

Questions began flying out of his mouth, "Why did that happen? Have you done that before? Was it hard getting the tube in? Do you think he will be alright?"

After I answered each of his questions I said, "Now it's my turn to ask you something."

"Ok, what?"

"How long do you figure it took me to get it in?" I asked, bracing for the worst. "Ten minutes … fifteen …twenty …?"

"*Minutes*?!" he asked, stunned. "Try forty-five seconds. Tops."

"You must be wrong," I said.

"I'm not. I looked at the clock the second you started cutting and the second you finished. It was less than sixty seconds. It was super-fast," he replied again, as confidently as if I had just asked him if gravity existed. "That's why I thought you had done it before."

Apparently, time *had* slowed down and waited for me. I had only imagined that I had taken too long. Although it felt good to hear, it didn't matter. The only thing that mattered was if Jesus woke up.

Half an hour later, I was still sitting at the nurses' station, flicking a pen around with my fingers, when Jesus's nurse walked over to us. "Dr. McPherson, there's a problem with your patient!"

My stomach sank. My worst fears were about to be confirmed. I looked up at her and noticed she was smiling, "Your patient is definitely awake! He woke up and was flailing his arms around. We explained to him what had happened, and he calmed down, but he's got some questions. Come take a look!" she said, joyfully.

I shot up and ran to the bedside. Sure enough, Jesus was sitting up in bed clearly awake. He couldn't talk with the breathing tube still in his neck, so his nurse had given him a white board to write on. I couldn't believe my eyes. Not only was he alive, but his brain had survived! I was overjoyed. I had never felt as happy in my life as I was in that moment.

As I drove home for the second time that night, I no longer cared about such trivialities as having missed dinner. I realized that this was the first time that *I* had ever truly saved someone's life. As general surgery resident, I had helped perform plenty of lifesaving operations, but that was just a part of my job. In those situations, I could easily have been replaced by any other general surgery resident and the outcomes would have been the same. But this was different. If *I* had not been there, it was possible (very likely in fact), that Jesus would not be alive. For the first time in my life, it had been my decisiveness, skills, and determination that had saved a life. This victory belonged to *me*. This was exactly what I had been training so hard for.

Suddenly, it felt like all of the sleepless nights, cancelled plans, crying girlfriend, missed trips home, pain, suffering, and mental anguish for the last five years, had been *for something*. The words that Dr. Moore had said to me years before ran through my mind, I was going to be a surgeon, and that was a big deal.

CHAPTER 22—How It Ends

I drove to the hospital for the last time in the wee hours of a Friday in June of 2020 blasting Blink-182's song *Anthem*. I felt the tires of my car pass over each familiar bump, massaging each curve in the road like I had thousands of times before. By now, I could do the entire drive with my eyes closed. Driving to work had always been my favorite part of the day. I loved cruising alone through the abandoned early-morning streets. Later they would be bustling with activity. But for now, I had the world to myself. My final moments of solitude for the rest of the day.

I pulled my car into the same spot I'd parked in for the last five years, but for the first time, I didn't consider going back home, getting back into bed, and going back to sleep. Every morning for five years, I'd sat in this spot wondering if I belonged, doubting my ability to finish residency, and constantly fighting back the urge to drive back home and go back to sleep. From intern year onward, my doubts grew and festered, culminating in the time I marched into Dr. Moore's office and told her that I was quitting. After that day, even though I soldiered on, these doubts remained in the back of my mind. They were always there, whispering to me. The doubts grew louder and louder when I was tired; with each mistake I made; every day off I didn't get; each time I was called back into the hospital, leaving my girlfriend behind to wonder if we could ever have a normal life together.

Since the first time I heard this voice in the back of my head during intern year, it never went away. It remained, loud and constant. On days when I was well-rested, I could keep it to a whisper, but it was always there, waiting

199

for a sleepless night so that it could strike, rising up from the shadows of my mind, and scream at me to quit, telling me that I shouldn't have ever even been there in the first place, that I wasn't good enough, that everything I had accomplished had been due to dumb luck, the fact that I had even gotten into medical school at all was a mistake, a mistake that my general surgery residency program had repeated. Somehow, I had fooled them all. My childhood friends' parents, through their unspoken words, had been right.

Occasionally, a victory at work—like saving Jesus's life—would quench the voice and leave me feeling confident that becoming a surgeon had been the right choice. But victories like those were few and far between, unfairly outnumbered by defeats like Kevin, Antonio, the Tanakas, and all of the burn patients waiting to be put back together again with cadaver skin. These constant ups and downs made me feel like I was on an endless emotional roller coaster.

For five years, I had wrestled between wanting more than anything to escape residency, yet not wanting to squander my good luck. I was convinced luck was the only reason I was even there in the first place. This juxtaposition of feelings would have kept me up at night ... if I hadn't been so tired.

At 7:45 a.m., I had just begun my final operation as a resident, a gallbladder removal. How fitting. It had been my first surgery as an intern, and it would be my last before graduation. As I injected numbing medicine into the sleeping patient's abdomen, I tented up the skin and remembered how I had cringed the first time I had done this. Over the years, my fear of blood had dissipated completely, the result of spending every waking hour in the hospital, O.R., and trauma bay. In other words, five years of being covered in blood had helped me get over my fear.

Dr. Yang stood across the operating room table from me and watched me. He loved to operate, and I knew that beneath his surgical mask, he was grinding his teeth and fighting back the urge to take my final operation away from me. Everything was going fine.

Dr. Yang and I stood in the surgeon's lounge after we finished operating for the day. I wasn't even on call. I would never again be on call here. It was time for me to go home to my girlfriend and cross the final "X" off my calendar.

Dr. Yang pulled off his surgical cap to reveal a head covered in white hair. He had been a surgeon for a long time, and he had seen enough to fill thousands of pages like these. Over the past five years, we had spent thousands of hours together, and this would be the last time we saw each other. We looked at each other in silence, unsure of what to say.

Eventually, Dr. Yang stuck out his hand and said, "You did a good job." We shook hands. I could count on one hand the number of compliments attendings had given me during residency, and I would still have four fingers left.

I smiled and thanked him.

Six hours later, I drove away from the hospital for the last time. For the first time, I finally felt free. I looked over at my phone sitting silently on the passenger seat of my car. I would never be called back again. Residency was over.

That night, we had a special dinner to celebrate my graduation from residency. My girlfriend and my parents were there—my mother, of course, beaming proudly, just like she had when I graduated med school five years earlier. I gave a brief speech, thanked everyone, and said my goodbyes. As cliché as it is to say, it was a bittersweet moment. Residency had been both exciting and traumatic, and I was relieved that it was over. But at the same time, I knew that with each second that passed, I would grow to miss it. Like all experiences in life, the bad memories would fade first and leave behind the good ones. Eventually, I would forget how tired I had always been, how badly I'd wanted to give up, the shame of being yelled at, or feeling like I would never make it. Instead, these memories would be permanently replaced with victories like Jesus, how *good* it felt to eat goldfish crackers from the cafeteria at two a.m., or what it was like to finally be told that I had done a "good job."

As I write this, I'm in California, where my adventure first began. It's four a.m., and in an hour, I'll be heading to the hospital. I woke up early to write this because this time of day is peaceful and still my favorite. The road outside my window is quiet, and from where I am sitting, I can hear the ocean waves crashing onto the sandy beach. But for the first time, in a long time, that is all I hear. The voice in the back of my head is finally gone. It disappeared when I graduated, and it never came back. That voice was my biggest enemy, and by not giving up, I defeated it. And perhaps *that* has been my greatest achievement.

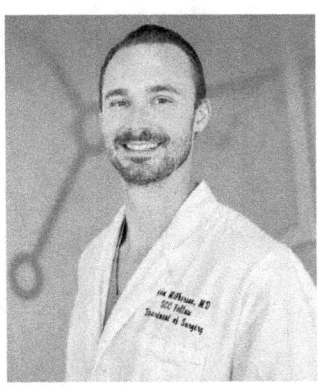

About the Author

Born in Southern California, Ryan McPherson is the first in his family to pursue a career in medicine. He attended medical school in Kansas City, Missouri. Afterward, he completed five years of general surgery residency in Phoenix, Arizona, followed by an additional year of fellowship training in trauma surgery in Los Angeles, California. At the time of this writing, he has been practicing for four years, and with each passing day, loves what he does more and more. He continues to work with residents and spends time discussing the rigors of training and burn out.

Keep In Touch

Dr. McPherson would love to hear from you! He regularly checks and responds to messages at:

RyanMcPhersonAuthor@gmail.com

Instagram: @Ryan_McPherson_Author